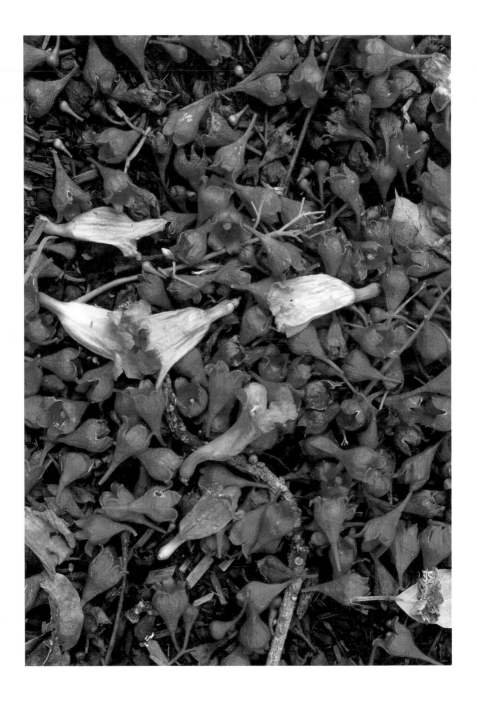

Praise for Georgia Blain

'Blain is a writer of such lucidity and strength that her characters speak, undeniably, for themselves … What makes it possible to contain tragedy in words, so that the reader enters into the experience and passes through it, cleansed? The Greek playwrights had their own answers to this question; but the question, I suspect, is far older than their version of it. Each generation of authors must find the right words for writing about death.'
DOROTHY JOHNSTON, *Sydney Morning Herald*

'Picking a favourite Georgia Blain novel is like picking a favourite child … Blain intelligently asks the big questions — about mortality, grief, forgiveness and how hard it can sometimes be to love those we're supposed to.'
North and South

'Blain writes enchantingly about the interstices of life, the places where morality and meaningfulness blur, and characters try to justify their actions or deal with their emotions … lyrical and lucid.'
Herald Sun

'Whenever I need reminding of the preciousness of ordinary life I return to this stunning novel of forgiveness and family, which gives clear, beautiful voice to the fierce luck of being alive.'
CHARLOTTE WOOD

'My favourite work of fiction in this year was Georgia Blain's lush and loss-ridden *Between a Wolf and a Dog*. It's a novel about the ways in which we hurt each other, or are hurt by the world, yet it is hopeful and redemptive in the small moments and minute joys that it charts.'

FIONA WRIGHT

'Many adjectives have been used to describe Georgia Blain's work, including evocative, powerful, atmospheric, haunting, rich, thought-provoking, skilful, uncompromising and finely detailed — all of which apply to this collection of short stories.'
Books+Publishing

'There's a quiet, understated quality to her prose, an introspection in her narrative that makes her words glow dully with slow-burning intensity … Relationships in all their combinations and permutations are skilfully dissected by an author with a keen eye and a firm grasp.'
THUY ON, *The Sun-Herald & The Age*

'Blain's achievement with the short story form is to render it a mid point between the overt artifice of fiction and the covert artifice of life-writing … her stories fill up with ambiguity … characterised by an irresolution that mimics the resistance of experience to shape and comprehension.'
STELLA CLARKE, *The Weekend Australian*

'Told with subtlety, tenderness and, skill, *The Secret Lives of Men* displays Georgia Blain's superb ability to convey both the joys and struggles of daily life and its impact on each of us. Blain is a gifted writer: through her storytelling we come to know ourselves better.'
TONY BIRCH

'[An] elegant, intelligent and affecting novel from a writer at the height of her powers.'
The Saturday Paper

'Heartfelt, wise, and emotionally intelligent, *Between a Wolf and a Dog* is a beautifully tender exploration of the complications of family love, self-knowledge, and the struggle for forgiveness.'
GAIL JONES, author of *A Guide to Berlin*

'Acute and finely detailed … [Blain's] refusal to disentangle and simplify is one of the strengths of this quiet, beautifully written and resonant memoir.'
BRENDA NIALL, *Sydney Morning Herald*

'An astute and intelligent observer, her insights make compelling reading. *Births Deaths Marriages* is a superbly crafted, richly layered, collection of beautifully written stories, one that readers are bound to return to again and again.'
Readings Monthly

THE MUSEUM OF WORDS

Scribe Publications
18–20 Edward St, Brunswick, Victoria 3056, Australia
2 John St, Clerkenwell, London, WC1N 2ES, United Kingdom

First published by Scribe 2017

Typeset in 11.8/17.85pt Adobe Garamond Pro by the publisher
Image placement Andrew G Taylor
All photographs and images copyright Andrew G Taylor, unless otherwise stated.
Extract from 'A Southern Rose' on p. 59 reprinted here with permission of Odessa Blain.

Printed and bound in China by 1010 Printing Asia Limited

Scribe Publications is committed to the sustainable use of natural resources
and the use of paper products made responsibly from those resources.

9781925322255 (Australian edition)
9781911344544 (UK edition)
9781925548389 (e-book)

CiP records for this title are available from the British Library
and the National Library of Australia.

scribepublications.com.au
scribepublications.co.uk

For my mother, Anne, my dear friend Rosie,
and the loves of my life, Andrew and Odessa

Foreword

I notice the date as I start writing, and realise it is only three months to the day since Georgia's death. It's not a long time by anyone's count. No wonder emotions are still raw.

Georgia was my life-partner, and we lived together for twenty years. She was diagnosed with brain cancer (Stage 4, Glioblastoma Multiforme) in November 2015, and died thirteen months later. Age fifty-one.

Georgia began writing *The Museum of Words* shortly after her diagnosis, and she finished a near-final draft just before she died. Knowing she was not long for this world, she mentioned the possibility of me writing an introduction, and I suggested we use some images at various places throughout the text. There was a loose consensus on both of these ideas, but that is about as far as we got.

Last night I printed out the manuscript, ready to continue editing today. Tears were rolling down my cheek before I got to the end of the first page. Georgia's voice was so fresh and clear — the words 'vibrant' and 'alive' spring to mind, but, of course,

there is something wrong with this picture.

As tender and painful as it was, once I started reading, I found it addictive. An old friend of mine, Junji, once described melancholy as the feeling of enjoying being sad. I can't say I enjoyed being sad, but I didn't want this feeling to stop.

Nonetheless, I forced myself to put the manuscript aside, determined to try and approach it fresh in the morning. I cleared my desk and other day-to-day work in preparation. I wanted a clear head, too. No drinking. (Well, only two glasses.)

I was woken by a dream, and then by a 4am-busy mind. Ideas for this introduction pinging and ricocheting around. In the dream, Georgia and I were sleeping outside, and, when it became light enough, I realised we were lying under trees full of blossom. Not just any blossom — cherry blossom. Below, a Japanese family were having a picnic breakfast in the park. I waved good morning, and a Japanese woman waved good morning back. Actually, I sang out 'ohayō' and she sang back the refrain 'gozaimasu' (it made perfect 'dream sense', but to literally translate, it would be something like I sang out 'good morning', and she sang back 'to be wishing you').

After our greetings, I enjoyed the slightly bizarre and uncharacteristic sight of Georgia running around and kicking a football, then gathering it and kicking it again. It was a park like Melbourne's Botanical Gardens, and Georgia was dressed in a purple dress, had long black hair, and looked like a ten-year-old Japanese girl. But I knew it was her, because shortly before leaving to kick the footy, she'd told me, still lying under

the cherry blossom, that I'd be the one who'd have to get up and go back to check on Odessa (our daughter). 'It doesn't matter if you are still half asleep and feeling tired — I haven't even had a coffee yet!'

In her last kick and chase, she was already at the place that she kicked the ball to. It was like a trick jump-cut edit in a film.

I first read a complete draft of *Museum of Words* the day before Georgia died. It was intense, but also compelling. Despite its disparate themes — words, language, Rosie, Anne, cancer, mortality — there was just such a strong, clear voice and through-line, like an arrow. What was, essentially, a first draft felt like it had written itself. The words flowed so easily. Of course, Georgia did have a particular clarity and skill as a writer, and a lifetime of reading and writing underlay this feeling of effortlessness. And, as Georgia points out in the pages to come, it would be hard to consciously script some of the circumstances surrounding the writing of this book. But Georgia was nothing if not disciplined. Early rise. Medication. Dog walk. Breakfast. More medication, meditation, coffee, and then one hour of power. Five hundred words later, here she comes.

One of the things Georgia recalls in the book is our time walking Odessa to kindergarten, when she was about four. During one of these walks, Odessa asked me, 'How fast is the speed of life?' It struck me as one of those innocent but poignant things that kids sometimes say. This was before the ubiquity of mobile phones and the emerging lexicon of mis-texts, so it also made an impression because of the closeness of 'light' and 'life'.

(And how did this four-year-old kid know enough to even ask about the speed of life / light?). I mention it now because the 'speed of life' took on a whole new meaning watching Georgia's mother's rapid decline with Alzheimer's, and Georgia's demise after her initial diagnosis.

I can't remember when Georgia felt the manuscript was solid enough to send to her editor at Scribe (Marika Webb-Pullman), but it must have been around the time of 11 September. This is one of two 'astrologically charged' dates that are mixed up with the end of Georgia's life. The first was 11 November 2015, the day she had brain surgery to remove as much of the tumour as possible. The other was ten months later: Sunday 11 September, the day of Georgia's second seizure. This date marked both the return of the brain tumour and the beginning of the end of her writing days. The speed of life can be very fast indeed.

Georgia sent Marika the manuscript for *Museum of Words* soon after this 9/11 date, and after a minor structural edit, Marika sent Georgia a marked-up copy of her manuscript, with suggested changes to accept or reject. I was copied in on this exchange, because by this stage, Georgia's health had become even more precarious, and she wanted me in on the dialogue between her and Marika, in case of a debilitating seizure or worse. Georgia being Georgia, the changes were mostly small — word repetition, that sort of thing. And Georgia had good faith in Marika's editorial skill from a previous working relationship. So much so, she was happy for me to work through Marika's marked-up editorial suggestions. (Yes, I was tempted to do a

few rewrites, and see if anyone would notice if I snuck in a few extra words, but somehow I didn't let the power go to my head, and resisted the imp of the perverse).

It was a family affair. I sat at the kitchen table with a laptop, working through Marika's suggestions. Georgia lay on a couch nearby, watching TV and chatting to Odessa. If there was any doubt, I ran suggestions past Georgia, but she seemed too fatigued in the end to really care. Or, at least, that is what I thought until I suggested replacing X with Y — and both she and Odessa firmly said, '*No, no, it definitely should be X*'.

I'm a filmmaker by trade and training, and so I feel like somewhat of an interloper here. That being said, the book-editing process is different to film, but it is not altogether foreign. The process Marika and I have been involved in is akin to fine-cutting a film. Technically speaking, a rough cut is locked off when all the storytelling elements are in an agreed place and order. It is then ready to be fine-cut. In this stage, every edit or cutting point in the film is examined and either left the same, or a few frames are added or taken away. A frame of film is $1/24^{th}$ of a second, so three frames here or there is only $1/8^{th}$ of a second. Not much. But the interesting thing is that this small amount can really make a cut 'work'. Suddenly, lumpy edits go 'pop'; turgid scenes become fluid; and overly jumpy, staccato transitions gain necessary pause and poetry. The right weight. The right measure.

I am telling you this here because although Georgia handed Marika something akin to a locked off 'rough cut', Marika then

did the 'fine cut'. She has made it flow. Made it zing.

Another change made to the original is that we have added images. Apart from the 'fine cut' and insertion of images, though, what you are reading here is, essentially, very similar to what I read the day before Georgia died.

This talk of editing and mortality reminds me of an existential flash I had many years ago when editing a documentary. I was a student at film school, and I was loving the process of editing a film that I had also directed. But Xmas and final assessment deadlines were approaching, and I was fast running out of time. This led to my revelation that this was what life would be like when our time came. We would try and make sense of it all, and create a beautiful, well-crafted whole, but probably it would be like my documentary: a few moments shining, but mostly of variable quality and a bit of a mess overall. *C'est la vie.*

Georgia's *Museum of Words* — unlike my film-school documentary — has the feeling of a work that is well resolved and complete. Reading it gives the impression that Georgia gained some satisfaction in making a sense of her life and work through writing this book. If this is the case — and I *do* think it is — it is particularly special that she was able to produce this book in the last year of her life.

But a book is not a life, and there is a horrifying randomness to someone so young and otherwise healthy being struck down by a disease that, statistically speaking, affects only 3 per 100,000 of a population.

Georgia's mother, Anne Deveson, features prominently in

these pages, as does her dear friend, Rosie Scott, and the book is as much a love letter to these two as it is a meditation on words, language, and writing. When Georgia finished this manuscript, she, Anne, and Rosie were all alive.

Anne died on Georgia's birthday, two days after Georgia (making 12 December, for me, another 'astrologically charged' date). As I write, Rosie is still alive, but she is in palliative care, being lovingly cared for by her immediate family.

So there is loss and a terrible sadness surrounding this creation. But it is a creation. Something new has come out of this sadness and loss. And this is a wonderful thing.

—AGT, *March 2017*

Looking back, I wish I had paid more attention to it; it was the only clue as to what was going to follow.

I remember telling several friends. 'There is something wrong with my words,' I would say.

I wasn't that alarmed — it was just that my speech wasn't quite right. I certainly wasn't worried enough to see a doctor, but I was concerned enough to remark on it several times.

Most of the time, the conversation would slide off into a discussion of forgetfulness, the inability to remember names, faces, and even places, as we reached our late forties and early fifties.

I had always prided myself on my memory, but I, too, had become someone who forgot.

Once, a friend of mine reminded me of a trip we'd made to Rome together.

We were having dinner at her house and reminiscing: tales of our youth, early loves and drunken nights.

I was confused. I was sure that the first and only holiday

I'd had in Rome was the visit I made in my early forties with my daughter, Odessa, and my mother, Anne. We went to visit Anne's brother, who spent half his time living in Trastevere, and the other half in Umbria, with a woman in each location.

My friend laughed in disbelief: how could I fail to remember the earlier trip I'd made with her, along with my boyfriend of the time, and a friend of ours, Russell? It wasn't until she took out a photo, the four of us sitting by the Spanish Steps, all eating gelati, that I realised I had been there before. And then the details came back. The hotel we had stayed in had a curfew, and we'd had to rush back each night to get in before the door was locked. My boyfriend and I were arguing terribly, on the brink of breaking up. I remembered the time he had shouted at me in a clothes shop and left in a temper. We'd been locked in battle about whether a neckline was square or round. Our friend Russell spent every day visiting a magician. He was trying to buy a levitation trick, and the magician had to know if he was worthy of the trick, if he could learn it and perform it faultlessly, before he would sell it to Russell.

How could I have forgotten all of that?

But each time the conversation drifted off into lapses of memory (my Rome story frequently trotted out to demonstrate — laughingly — just how bad I was), I knew that this problem with my words wasn't just forgetfulness. It was something else.

At the time, I was under a lot of stress.

My mother was in her eighties and had recently been diagnosed with Alzheimer's. I was the only child in Sydney

and I felt very responsible for caring for her. I wanted to fix everything, and I ran around getting rosters in place, cleaners, sorting her money, wrangling her friends, all of who were eager to help.

She resisted, usually by pretending that she would get better, sometimes by actively dismantling the care I had set up. By nine o'clock most mornings, I had fielded at least a dozen phone calls from people who had no idea what was going on in this sea of frequently changing arrangements.

For the past fifteen years, she had lived in a converted shop by the beach, which she'd painted yellow with a bright-orange door. The shopfront was her office, a huge book-lined room with an old shearer's table in the middle. Like me, she was a writer.

She wrote three books in that house — one a novel, the other on resilience, and the last on peace, just before her official diagnosis.

She and I were very different. I was more introverted, more organised, and so terrified of deadlines that I usually got projects done months ahead of the due date.

She was gregarious, loved people, ignored deadlines, read drafts of her work to friends in cafés, and frequently drove editors and publishers to pull out their hair.

However, this last book of hers was more troubled than most.

She just couldn't seem to get it done. She printed out draft after draft, always on yellow paper (she loved yellow paper). Sometimes, she told me it was 35,000 words; sometimes, 170,000. Footnotes and references were frequently lost, hard

drives crashed, she was convinced that a 'rogue font' had got into her computer, manuscripts were couriered back and forth from Melbourne to Sydney in an attempt by the publishers to wrangle the project by putting it into hard copy, but old drafts got mixed in with the new.

She became distressed, sometimes even angry, each time I tried to broach the topic of the book.

It was like she had forgotten how to write, but it wasn't the words that eluded her; it was all the building blocks that she had once had at her command, the way in which a book is put together, that had gone missing.

All writers struggle with this at times. But with Anne and this last book, it was as though each time she assembled it, a pernicious wind swept all the pages up again, flying them to each corner of the house, out on the street, and she had to run around frantically trying to gather them.

I know now that this was the first evidence of Alzheimer's. At the time I was suspicious; I think she was, too.

After the book came out, and she had finished publicising it, she finally agreed to do tests. The results were not good.

As I write this in my room, also book-lined, I am curious as to how long ago the publication date actually was. I get up and find a copy of it. I only have one, whereas I have so many copies of her other books.

Waging Peace, by Anne Deveson.

I look to the date and I am shocked that it was only three years ago.

4

Our lives have changed so much since then.

She is now in a nursing home and rarely leaves her bed. She knows us still, but she doesn't really know what is wrong with me.

Just after I got her into care, I was diagnosed with an aggressive brain tumour, first signalled by something going awry with my own words. And it was not forgetfulness.

As I type this I am aware that I have hit my limit — about an hour of the intense focus and concentration necessary to assemble sentences on a page, and I am done in. Nothing is making much sense anymore. It is like the cotton in the branches of the cottonwood trees, the trees that line the river in the park at the bottom of the hill where I live.

Each spring this cotton forms, floating away in the breeze, wafting, insubstantial, and always so maddeningly out of reach.

———

The problem with my words was hard to define. I knew it wasn't just forgetfulness, an inability to lay my hand on the right word. The technical term for it is dysphasia, which is simply an impairment of language, sometimes called aphasia, although aphasia is, strictly speaking, a total inability to form language or speech. Language is controlled by the left-hand side of the frontal lobe, and this is where my tumour was located.

Strangely, I learnt all this a month or so before my own tumour made itself undeniably evident with a total global seizure. My dearest friend, Rosie, a writer as well, was also diagnosed with a brain tumour, glioblastoma multiforme (GBM) Stage

4, some weeks before my own diagnosis. Her tumour sat, as mine sat, right in the language centre of her brain. Before her diagnosis, she too had dysphasia, which took the form of frequently saying the wrong word, although it was often closely related to the thing she was trying to say.

It is hard to believe, that we would both go down with the same thing.

If this were fiction, I would say it was too far-fetched.

But unfortunately, it is true.

I had known Rosie for over twenty years. Too young to be my mother, and too old to be my sister, she was nevertheless like family. Rosie was one of the first people I told when I was pregnant, when Anne was diagnosed with Alzheimer's, when I felt despair at my writing, and when I felt joy.

A lot of people feel like that about her. She is perhaps one of the most loved and cherished people I know.

Rosie was in France on holiday when her speech broke down. I saw her just before she left, and I knew there was something wrong. She seemed anxious about going. She'd been tired, working on anthologies about the Northern Territory intervention and also doing a lot of projects with asylum seekers. This work usually fired her, but she seemed to be struggling. I knew she'd wanted to get back to her own novels for a long time, but had been unable. She'd lost some of her joy in writing, and she was hoping that this holiday would perhaps kickstart her own work. I thought she was worried that going away wouldn't reignite her. Perhaps she was depressed; but Rosie

never liked to talk about her own problems.

We had Indian takeaway in her lounge room, and I knew she was avoiding any mention of her own troubles. She repeated herself, her speech cautious as she tried to find the right words. She questioned me, as she often did — about my writing, Anne's Alzheimer's, my partner, Andrew — but she didn't seem to listen to the answers.

When Rosie arrived in France, her daughter (who was in Sydney) called me to tell me she was worried about her. Rosie could barely speak. She kept confusing words. She also couldn't write — a simple email was riddled with spelling mistakes and grammatical errors.

Rosie's daughter wanted to bring her home.

On her return she had a brain scan, and they discovered the tumour.

I remember being totally floored by the news. I sat in my car and wept, inconsolable. How could I cope without Rosie?

A few days later, she went into surgery. I visited her in the hospital as soon as she was out of intensive care. Her head was shaved, and she could barely speak. The speech pathologist had given her a board that she could use to point to 'yes' or 'no', and that she could also use to spell words.

She kept swiping it away in frustration, trying to talk, only ever managing to run two or three words together. I sat by her side, and I am ashamed to say I cried.

As she recovered from the operation, her speech returned. She was not as verbally dexterous as she once was, and when

she became tired, what ability she had would crumble, but in those early weeks she always had enough words to make herself understood. Once, when I visited her at home, she told me that her husband and daughters had gone to see 'trouble'. I knew they were seeing the oncologist — they'd told me — and her choice of this word made perfect sense.

Before I, too, was diagnosed, I occasionally confused words — many people do. I would tell Andrew to put the dishes in the fridge, rather than the dishwasher. I noticed I was doing this a bit more than usual, but I put it down to the stress of trying to get Anne into a home, and on top of that, what was happening to Rosie.

But I was always aware that there seemed to be an additional problem. It was as though the building blocks of my sentences, so much that we say without even thinking about the words we are choosing, had gone. I had to think. About every clause. At times, I was self-conscious about my lack of fluency.

Even then, with what had happened to Rosie, I didn't pay much attention to the affliction. It was too ridiculous to contemplate that I had the same cancer in the same spot. And unlike Rosie, my communication was still largely intact. I was writing, and no one seemed to notice any difficulties when I talked, despite my own awareness of something being not quite right.

It was about two weeks after I finally got Anne into a home, and about four weeks after Rosie's operation, that I collapsed on a bed of jacaranda and flame-tree blossoms, my body jerking,

blood frothing at my mouth.

I didn't see this. Andrew and Odessa, my seventeen-year-old daughter, did.

The last thing I remembered was mowing the lawn, and the intensity of the colours — the emerald-green grass, the cut-glass sky, the white tufts of cloud — and then I came to in the back of an ambulance.

The man sitting next to me told me I'd had a seizure and they were taking me to emergency, and then started asking me questions. What was my name? Where did I live? What date was it? Who was the Prime Minister of Australia?

I couldn't answer him.

Not because I didn't understand the questions — it was because I didn't know the answers, and even if I had known, the words wouldn't come.

Andrew was in the front seat next to the ambulance driver. They were chatting about the electric lawnmower I had been using.

'How ya finding the Ozito?' the driver asked.

I tried to laugh, to tell him that Andrew would have had no idea; I was the one who mowed the lawn.

Once again, I couldn't utter a sound.

In the emergency department, I began to be able to form simple responses to questions. They were scattered like pebbles, and I had to strain to reach them — my name, where I was. The date was harder to reach, and the Prime Minister was impossible.

I don't remember much about the hours I spent there.

I know there were scans and visits by doctors who were at first circumspect about what had caused the seizure, but who then began to break the news to me. It seemed there was a tumour, about the size of a golf ball; it was sitting on my front left lobe, it appeared to be aggressive, I would have to be admitted. I would need surgery.

Each time I stretched out my fingers to hold on to hope, it was snatched away.

In the cubicle next to me there was a woman of about sixty. I think she was there with one of her children. She pressed a small crochet cross into the palm of my hand, and told me she would pray for me. 'This will bring you luck,' she said. 'You will be alright.'

I am not normally superstitious or religious, but I still have the cross, all these months later. It sits on my desk, near the base of my computer.

I am inordinately wary of losing it.

I was operated on about a week after I was admitted. By then, my command of language had returned to the same state it was in before. Slightly troubling, but the complete loss (even if only for a brief time) put it into perspective. As did the fact that, ultimately, the tumour was incurable. They would blast it with chemotherapy and radiation, but it would return. It was probable that I wouldn't last more than a couple of years.

As I signed the consent forms for the operation, the surgeon told me there was a two per cent risk that my ability to communicate would be lost. He said I might come out of

THE MUSEUM OF WORDS

surgery unable to talk or write.

Two per cent was low.

(On the flip side, the chances of surviving up to five years were also two per cent, but I clung on to that.)

I didn't ask him whether I would be able to comprehend language, nor did I really contemplate what it would mean to be without words. I was clinging on to life, willing to buy whatever time I could.

I always wanted to be a writer. I cannot remember a time when I didn't. It began as soon as Anne started telling me stories, followed by her reading them to me (which she did from a very young age).

I wasn't yet in school when I first cracked the code: when the lines became letters, and the letters became words, and I was able to read for myself.

I was sitting on the floor of my older brother's room, looking at the books in his bookshelves. I was four; Jonathan was seven. He wouldn't have been in there with me; he didn't like me coming into his room, but I often snuck in when he was downstairs or out playing with friends.

There was dark-blue sisal matting on the floor, scratchy on my bare skin, and the sunlight was streaming in through the huge arched windows. His bed was wooden — convict made, my parents told us — and always tidy. In fact, the whole room was immaculate. My father, who was obsessive-compulsive, ensured all of our rooms were kept that way. I didn't find it

onerous (I was very adept at the neat surface), but Jonathan was frequently in trouble for mess.

I took an edition of Grimm's fairytales out of one of the lower shelves. It had a yellow-and-grey cover and had boring black-and-white line drawings, scattered sparsely throughout. I liked pretending I could read, flipping through the pages, retelling myself the story in whatever words I chose.

But on that day, it began to make sense.

At first, it was just simple words: 'and', 'but'. Soon, I began to sound out more complex ones. I wanted to see if it was just that book, or all the others, that I was capable of decoding. I took them out excitedly, a pile soon forming around me.

I write as though my reading suddenly happened, but it would have been after years of bedtime stories, of following the words, without knowing I was following them, of time alone with Anne — and if I try hard I can almost remember her smell, warm wool, rich and soft, as I nestled in next to her. Just before Anne moved into the nursing home, we found the books she'd kept from our childhood, the Grimm's fairytales among them. There were also Ant and Bee books, simple illustrations in beautiful primary colours, the pages often scrawled on or torn by one of us (my father wouldn't have liked that at all); books by Maurice Sendak; and a whole series of Orlando, the marmalade cat. I liked the illustrations in those, but the stories were dull. Orlando was handsome, but insufferably boring.

'I can read,' I told Anne as I ran down the stairs that day. 'I can read.'

I opened a page, pointed to one of the easier words, and told her what it was. I found another, and then another.

She was impressed and delighted, but to me it was a miracle. This was a door that had opened to a secret garden, and it was mine.

I became a pain in the arse, taking more and more complex words to class, boasting that I could spell them and writing them up on the blackboard. I particularly remember being very proud of myself when I spelt 'catastrophe' without a mistake.

I was voracious, reading everything in Jonathan's room, soon graduating to the lounge room where books like Charmian Clift's *Peel Me a Lotus* appealed to me immensely, primarily because of the title (what was a lotus?), and others, more salacious, were read in secret.

At the same time, I began to make up stories of my own — horse stories, boarding-school stories, sometimes written down with pen and paper, sometimes just muttered to myself as I bounced my netball up and down the garden path, driving everyone crazy.

———

Anne, too, had always wanted to write, but she felt great unease with defining herself as an author; embarrassed, as though she was not worthy of the title.

In the clean-up of her house, we found all of her passports. I was a couple of months post surgery at this stage, and well into a gruelling schedule of treatment. For six weeks, I had daily radiation and chemotherapy. I then had a month break,

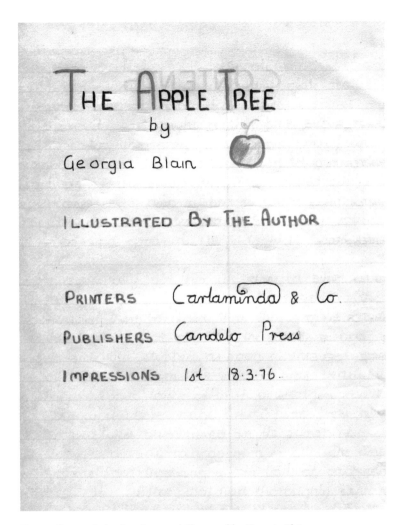

THE APPLE TREE
by
Georgia Blain

ILLUSTRATED BY THE AUTHOR

PRINTERS   Carlaminda & Co.
PUBLISHERS Candelo Press
IMPRESSIONS 1st   18.3.76.

Excerpt from early book written and illustrated by Georgia Blain

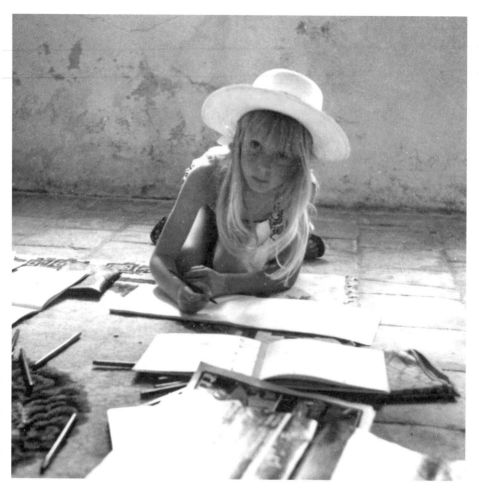

Georgia Blain, c. 1971

and then my chemotherapy dose was doubled, and given at less frequent intervals, for a further six months.

In the midst of this, we transferred Anne from respite care to permanent care. We had to trick her, to lie to her, to tell her that she would be going home as soon as she got stronger, and at first I hated it, but soon I became hardened to it as I tried to cope with my own illness.

We met a real estate agent, and gave ourselves a couple of months to clean up the house before we put it on the market. No one told her what we were doing — she would have been adamant that she didn't want the house sold — but we had to do it to pay for her room in the nursing home.

She was a hoarder, albeit organised (although the organisation had become increasingly frayed at the edges as the dementia got worse). She had kept *everything*: trunks of cloth that she wanted to make into dresses, all our childhood drawings, party invitations, hand-drawn cards from us, every bill, and, of course, every passport that she'd ever had.

I was tired to the bone, deeply despairing, and trying to keep myself from being overwhelmed by sorrow. It was too much for me, and I wanted to throw everything away. Fortunately, Andrew and a good friend, Murphy, were there to help. Each time I dragged something to the skip, they would look twice, surreptitiously pocketing anything that seemed worth keeping. They are hoarders, too, but now, as I sit with each of my mother's passports on my desk, I am glad that they didn't obey me when I told them to chuck it all, all of it.

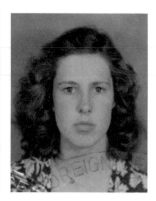

DESCRIPTION SIGNALEMENT		Wife-Femme
Profession Profession	*JOURNALIST*	
Place and date of birth Lieu et date de naissance	*Kuala Lumpur* *British Malaya* *19 June 1930.*	
Residence Résidence	*England*	
Height Taille	*5 ft 9½ in*	ft. in.
Colour of eyes Couleur des yeux	*Hazel*	

Details Anne Deveson passport, issued c. 1946

Anne's first passport lists her occupation as 'Student', crossed out, the word 'Journalist' written above it. (It's hard to believe that you were once able to strike a line through words on official identity documents.) She is twenty-one, about to embark on travels across Europe, with long, curly hair, and a strong and sensual face, and she's staring straight into the camera.

She told me she had studied science at university in the U.K. and was miserable. After a year she dropped out, taking to her bed and becoming increasingly overweight. Eventually she emerged, finding a job with a freelance journalist, Barbara Wace, who lived in a tiny bedsit on Fleet Street.

She loved it. This was what she was meant to do.

The next passport also lists her occupation as 'Journalist', and then, when she changes her name to Anne Blain, after marrying my father and coming to live with him in Australia, she becomes 'Broadcaster'.

The last passport, when occupation was still required to be

listed, categorises her as a 'Writer'. She had also gone back to her maiden name.

I am not sure how she would define herself now, if she were in her right mind and able to know what was being asked of her. I hope she would say 'Author', proudly.

———

We gave all the passports to Odessa.

Anne always felt Odessa was just like her, and she was so proud of her, frequently boasting of her achievements to anyone who would listen.

In some ways they are alike. They are both intrinsically shy but always wanting to challenge themselves, particularly through travel. Odessa hates being complacent. She is toying with the idea of also being a journalist when she finishes university. And so the passports were a fitting gift. But I am wary about drawing too many comparisons. Odessa is her own person, most of her life is in front of her, and she could change tack — perhaps voluntarily, perhaps by necessity.

I gather up all the passports and take them back to Odessa's room, aware that once again, I have come to an end. The words are floating. Two days ago, I completed another round of chemo. It not only makes me unbelievably tired (fatigue doesn't do justice to the sensation), but it also blurs my thoughts. It is like I am seeing with glasses that don't have the right prescription. I am no longer capable of the sustained effort at the desk that I once was. They call it 'chemo brain', a term I hate. It reminds me of when

I was pregnant and breastfeeding, a time during which mothers are often told that they won't be as on the ball as they used to be.

I shouldn't hate it. I should accept that I am weaker than I used to be, but I just don't want it pointed out to me — just as Anne initially baulked at me telling her she was getting older, she had dementia, and of course she couldn't do what she used to do.

Like mother, like daughter.

When I came out of surgery after the removal of my tumour, I was in the hushed, underground world of the ICU. An elderly Chinese nurse gave me sips of water and encouraged me to eat. She called me sweetie and washed me down with brisk but kind efficiency. I couldn't stop crying.

Andrew and Odessa sat by my side. They told me I was doing fine.

It was hard to speak.

Sometime later, I woke to see the surgical team by my bedside. They said the operation was a success. They had removed as much of my tumour as was visible. They were full of good cheer, too bright for the subdued world of intensive care.

I tried to reply, but my words were halting, difficult to hold on to.

'It's early days yet,' one of the doctors told me. 'There's been trauma.'

Andrew tried to reassure me by saying that my sentences were only a bit slower and slightly slurred. They would be bound to improve. The doctors recommended a speech pathologist and an occupational therapist, who would both visit me on the ward.

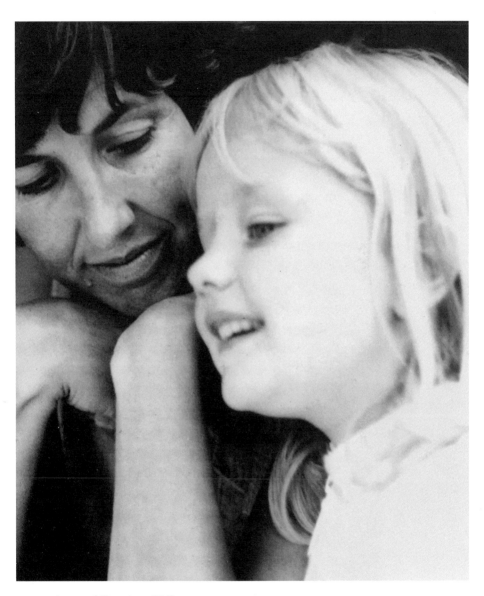

Anne and Georgia, c. 1970

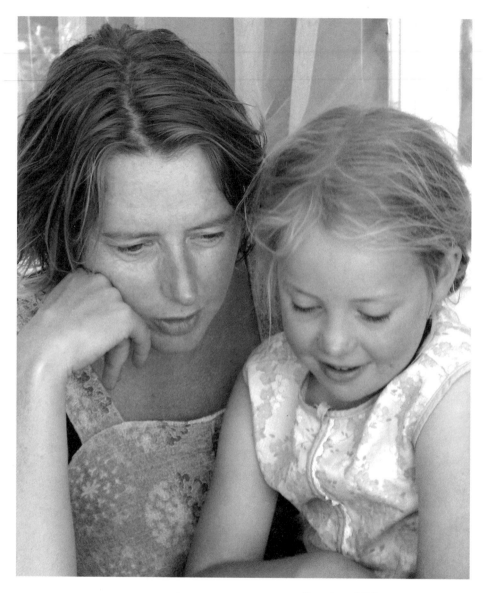

Georgia and Odessa, c. 2005

I met the occupational therapist in a makeshift exercise/storage room. She asked me if I would mind running through a few questions with her, just basic ones. They were similar to the ones that Anne had had to answer when she was diagnosed with Alzheimer's: fill in the numbers on the clock face; draw this shape; remember a sequence of words and later you'll be asked to repeat them back for me; count backwards in multiples of seven. She used to hate doing those tests. Once, she even cheated, writing down the season, the month, and the day on her arm, which I hoped would score extra points for ingenuity.

My brain was tired. I failed miserably at the clock face (strange how a clock face is still a part of these tests; I wonder whether anyone younger than me would be capable of drawing one). I also had trouble with the simple arithmetic, but my memory was fine. The woman assured me my results were normal, considering my surgery.

The speech pathologist came to my bedside. She was young and softly spoken.

Initially, she asked me to name objects that she held up for me — a pen, a cup, a watch — then she gave me cards with illustrated scenarios on them. They were old-fashioned, like the 'learn to read' books I'd had in my childhood: a woman in a frock doing the dishes, while outside her husband is pulling up in the driveway, a cat about to dart across the path of the car.

She asked me what was happening.

No, I tried to say. *This isn't the problem.* But I obeyed, spelling out the story for her.

Then she asked me to name all the words that I could think of beginning with 'F'.

All I could think of was 'Fat fuck', a term of abuse I'm ashamed to say I'd once used on a man after a heated exchange when he'd kicked my dog.

I couldn't think of any other words.

She tried various letters of the alphabet — each was only slightly better.

But still I didn't think this was getting anywhere near the heart of the issue. She assured me my vocabulary would improve, and I believed her. Even in those early days, I already had enough words at my command; I was able to duck and dart when the right word didn't come to mind immediately. I was nowhere near my full power, but I had enough.

Again, I was reminded of my mother. As her Alzheimer's progressed, I was amazed at how she remained verbally agile, weaving stories, fishing out words from the recesses of her mind, always wanting approval — 'that was a good word,' she would say — and even having a passable command of her schoolgirl Latin and French, which she loved to show off to Odessa.

I tried to articulate what was going on. The filing cabinets in my brain, the ones that contained the building blocks of sentences, were scrambled. I now had to hunt for the right clause, the right tense, whereas once they were all there, at my command, without having to think.

But even that didn't quite get to the nub of it. I became particularly stressed when I had to issue instructions, or plan.

I knew what should happen next in my head, but the words started to crumble away.

The speech pathologist told me that I should try and articulate chains of actions. How would I make a cup of tea? Every step of the way.

I didn't drink tea. Never have.

Remembering both Odessa and Anne, who loved tea, I tried to explain how to make a pot. It wasn't hard, but the speech pathologist was kind and didn't make me particularly stressed, which certainly helped.

Saying that the language centre is in the front left of the brain is a bit like saying Australia is in the southern hemisphere. It doesn't give you all that much information about Australia itself, a land that encompasses so much: deserts, cities, beaches, country towns. It is only if you zoom in that you'll get the finer details, the stuff that matters.

MRI technology is constantly improving (although, as my oncologist regularly reminds me, it is still far from an exact science), and work is being done on mapping out which areas of the brain affect which parts of our speech. The shape of the trauma, the size and location are all important, and all interrelated. Like real estate, however, location is of fundamental importance. The effect of damage to one brain region is dependent on whether or not other parts of the brain are also damaged — just like the effect of a fractured thumb will depend on whether or not the fingers are also fractured.

I knew, and still know, that my capacity to cope with stress

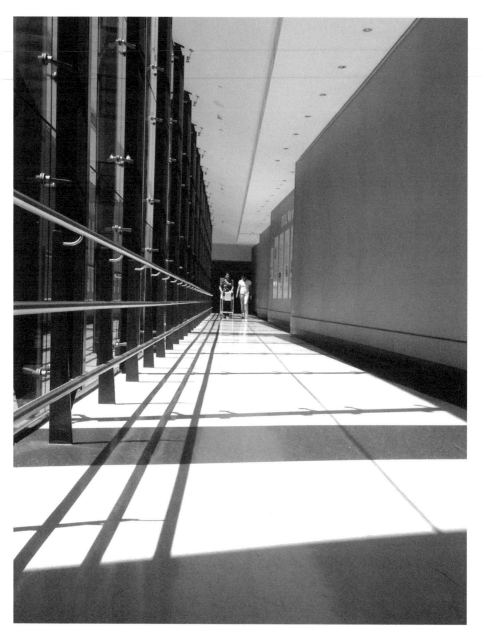

Corridor leading to MRI facility, RPA Hospital, November 2015

has been considerably lowered. It impacts on my ability to think logically, and also to speak. It is order that has been disarrayed.

But in retrospect, I think my distress was not commensurate with the affliction I was suffering. Even at the time, I was aware of this. It was just that what had already happened to my friend, Rosie, had made me wary about what could happen, how much worse my speech could get — and who would I be without words?

I only write in the morning. I have learnt that my brain is better earlier in the day. Steroids and two cups of strong coffee usually clear the fog.

I start by editing what I have done the day before, and I am always dismayed to see how convoluted and strained my expression gets as I near the end of the hour's writing done the previous day. I miss words. Clauses are jumbled. Was I always like this on a first draft, or have I become significantly worse? Will it improve when the side effects of the chemotherapy wear off? Will I ever be off chemotherapy? Will I have a period when I can write as though I am flying again?

Interestingly, I find I am reading more than ever.

During my late forties, I stopped reading books. I was working several jobs, trying to write, looking after Anne, and in the evening I wanted television series, social media — it would take a lot for a novel to hold my attention.

Odessa could occasionally drag me back. Like me when I was younger, she reads all the time. Unlike me, she took a

while to get the knack, but when she did there was no stopping her. There is still no stopping her. She is at sea without a book on the go.

By the time she reached high school, her tastes were adult, and she wanted me to share her appreciation of writers she discovered. Steinbeck was the first she urged me to re-read — *The Grapes of Wrath*. As a school student I had found it heavy going, earnest, depressing, the sheer grind of its hopelessness wearing me down. I wanted joy. Even a drop. But I took out my dog-eared copy, covered in plastic, with pencilled comments in the margins, accompanied by the occasional florid doodle. I started reading. It was a hurricane of rage, blistering, and that last scene — how stripped back, how elemental it is. I closed the book, all air gone out of my lungs, absolutely exhausted by its force.

She also wanted me to read Faulkner, a writer whom I had avoided at school. She told me she'd had to read *As I Lay Dying* twice before it made sense, and on my first and only reading, I pestered her constantly, trying to decipher who was doing what and who was related to whom.

But then the prose took over, the gothic horror of that corpse being dragged across the country, the poverty, again the hopelessness, and again that last scene — that last scene.

I will love a book forever if the final pages mark my subconscious.

Just before the tumour made itself evident with a seizure, I had found two authors, both working on similar but different

projects, whose work absorbed me totally — Karl Ove Knausgård and Elena Ferrante.

Both skirt the line between fiction and memoir. Knausgård is put more firmly in the autobiographical category, Ferrante in the fiction, although as she is presumably a woman, many readers assume her writing is close to her own life.

Knausgård's epic six-parter, grouped under the name 'My Struggle', plays with the inherent fictionalisation in all memoir. How do we remember the minute details of a child's birthday party: whom we spoke to in the kitchen, the staleness of the biscuits, all the prosaic details that make up life? His total absorption in the self (who would write a six-part memoir?) is also, presumably, a wry comment on a writer's total absorption in the self, grandiose and overblown to the extreme. And perhaps it's not just writers who can be accused of this — we all can be.

Ferrante's Neapolitan novels document a young girl growing up in post-war Naples, becoming educated, and a writer, ultimately escaping the poverty of her childhood, but never the mesh of relationships that ensnare and hold her there.

These are novels about the importance of feminism and education, but at the heart of them is the friendship between Elena and Lila. Elena obsesses over Lila; she observes her every move, constantly measuring her own worth in relation to her friend and finding herself wanting, despite being ultimately more successful. Lila, on the other hand, remains opaque, seen only through the prism of Elena's obsession.

I had started the last of Ferrante's series just before I had my seizure, and I finished it when I was in hospital. In fact, I finished the final instalment an hour before I went into surgery, the last chapter rushed through, barely leaving an impression. It was hard trying to read through the fear. Often, whole pages made little sense, the words wafting away — not because of the tumour itself, but because of all that I was trying to deal with. I felt like I wasted the last book, but I don't ever want to go back to it. It brushes too close to the anxiety and sorrow of that time. But it was the whole project that mattered, not the end, and I knew I had met, in Elena, a woman who felt the same unease in family (for different reasons) that I did. Both Knausgård and Ferrante make art of the everyday, the ordinary. As a writer, it fascinates me. The details of a dress, the alcohol you bought for a party, your teenage desperation to lose your virginity — how do you make it so engaging?

This is a project that I, too, attempt, whether I am writing fiction or memoir. This is what I try and grapple with: holding the ordinary up as a mirror to let us examine ourselves. As I look back on my work, I know that so much of what I have written is about the intricacies of family relationships; about distrust; guilt; corrosive anger; dependency. I have written my life over and over again (many writers do), seeking out commonality of experience with my characters, perhaps trying to affirm that I am not as unlikeable or uncharitable as I fear I am. Surely everyone is like that?

When I look back, it was strange that I didn't worry about

my capacity to comprehend post the operation — about the possibility of having reading torn away from me, or being unable to understand people when they were speaking to me. That concern never entered my mind. I was only worried about my capacity to communicate, about not being able to make myself understood.

I have since learnt that *comprehension* of language is located in another part of the brain — still on the left side, but at the back rather than the front. Impairment produces receptive aphasia. Sufferers can formulate sentences without any grammatical errors, but they cannot convey the meaning of what they have just uttered. Sometimes, they also use meaningless words, nonsensical grammar, and unnecessary phrases that can make their speech incomprehensible.

It seems the two would have to be inextricably linked — how can you express yourself if you're not aware of meaning? It is like the serpent consuming its tail — each time I try to comprehend what it means, I go round and round in circles, ending up with nothing at all, or with a sentence like Chomsky's example of a grammatically correct, but semantically nonsensical, sentence: *Colourless green ideas sleep furiously.*

———

Soon after I returned home from hospital, one of Rosie's daughters picked me up so that I could visit Rosie. She warned me that Rosie's speech wasn't fluent, but she assured me that her comprehension was absolutely fine.

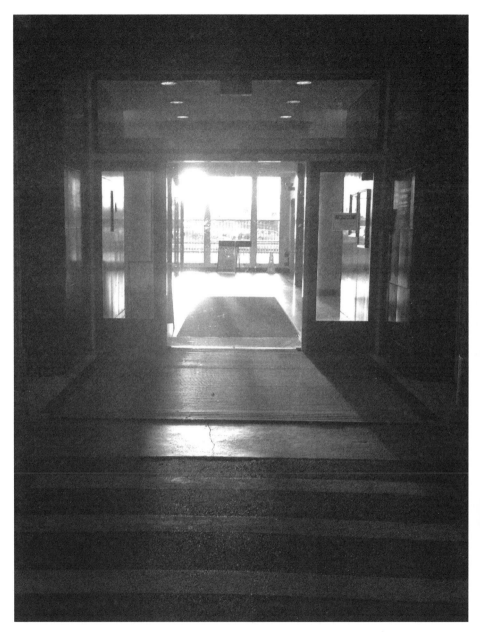

Sun setting at Camperdown Hospital, the evening before Georgia's brain surgery

At that time, Rosie was living in her inner-city flat while she was undergoing radiation treatment, and going up to her husband's in the Blue Mountains on the weekends.

It was early summer — crisp blue skies and still just enough freshness in the breeze to make the heat bearable. Her lounge room faced north, looking out on a majestic gum, silvery, like satin in the sunlight.

Rosie's speech was quite good, although as she became tired the words became harder to find.

We didn't speak about our respective tumours. Her family had warned me that she became stressed speaking about the illness, and she certainly seemed to want to slide off any mention of it. It was strange to be sharing this experience and not talking of it. But perhaps the nature of a life-threatening disease makes you separate out from other people, and you are alone in it. Words are frequently inadequate, but during that afternoon, she occasionally held my hand, rubbing it with her own, and looking into my eyes. We both knew what the other was going through.

We spoke about friends, writing, and books — books we'd loved, books we didn't like (despite the weight of popular opinion being against us), and books we wanted to read. She was judging an award and she had cartons of recent fiction and memoir. I took half a dozen home with me, on her recommendation.

That was probably the last relatively fluent conversation I had with her. Soon after, her language worsened (although it

wasn't always a straight decline — sometimes it would pick up again) and she stopped reading anything other than the odd article in the newspaper. I don't know whether it no longer held any joy for her, or whether it was a part of her brain that no longer functioned in the way it once had. I can't help but wonder whether this will be the way my tumour progresses, whether this pleasure that I have had for so long will be torn away from me.

About two years ago, Anne also began to find it too difficult to read.

Odessa, who was then almost sixteen, went with Anne and me on a holiday to Bali, shortly before Anne was diagnosed with Alzheimer's. I was filled with trepidation as to whether Anne would cope with a change of environment and jet lag, but friends urged me to go, saying I would be thankful later.

It was stressful. Anne wandered, frequently getting lost, unable to even find her way from her room to ours (we were in the room next door). We put notes in her pockets and bag, stating her name and where she was staying. She walked up and down the esplanade, making promises to all the women with clothes stalls that she would return and get a dress, and, with no idea of money, the sums she agreed to were hugely inflated. Every time I took a morning walk, these women would hold out clothing and call out: 'for your mother.' Eventually, she sprained her ankle and had to be in a wheelchair. It was like being with a child again — we had to take turns looking after her.

Each day we sat in the lush gardens, cooling ourselves off in

the pool. Brightly coloured wooden fishing boats were pulled up onto the beach; families swam while women lazily tried to sell massages, soon giving up in the heat. Anne and Odessa read *The New York Times*. Sometimes, Anne would complete an article, but often she folded the paper after a few minutes, closing her eyes. When she awoke, she returned to the same story, never finishing it.

She was also reading Ann Patchett's *State of Wonder*. I had lent it to her five months previously, exhorting her to read it, just like Odessa does to me. One day, she was on page 10; the next day, she was on page 227; the day after that, page 152.

She always insisted that she was reading it from front to back (her Alzheimer's was still undiagnosed then, but I am ashamed to think I even queried her), but both Odessa and I knew that the narrative was lost to her. She could only read small sections at a time, and there was no order to them at all.

Now, she doesn't even try to read — papers, cards from friends, poetry, let alone books. She also doesn't watch television, nor does she listen to the radio. She lies in her bed, often with her eyes closed, complaining of the buzzing in her head.

It was almost summer when I came out of hospital.

I had pamphlets on how to cope with cancer, all written in reassuring plain English, careful to avoid terms like 'battle' or 'fight'. I was living with cancer. Living with the constraints that inevitably come with illness.

I also had sheets from the speech pathologist, with exercises. *What would you do if you went to a restaurant and there was a fly in your soup?* No, it wasn't a joke. Step by step, I was meant to tell Andrew what I would do.

I refused to play the game.

'Not eat it,' I said.

After about day two, I put the sheets in a drawer and forgot about them.

It was unseasonably warm, and when our air conditioner broke down, I tried to explain to various service men what the problem was and the steps I'd already taken to try to narrow down the fault. I often had to write the conversation down. It was incredibly difficult. I felt as though my speech was impaired

to the same extent as if I were trying to dress myself with one hand tied behind my back.

I also had to have meetings with insurance companies and superannuation agents. They were all men, well trained in being caring but not too invasive, and they were kind. They knew it was hard for me to constantly fill out forms explaining that I was likely to be dead in the next sixteen months. But they didn't know that it was even more challenging for me to be unable to articulate my needs in conversations such as these, with the same ease I'd once had. I could talk about my diagnosis, I could even talk about dying, but talk of legal and financial details were hard. I frequently became tongue-tied, embarrassed, afraid of being thought of as stupid or brain-damaged.

I was also determined to write. In the first six weeks, I documented my days, amassing more than 20,000 words. Sometimes, I was awash with sorrow and grieving. Other times, there was a saturated hue, an intensity that I'd never felt before. I was leaving the world, crossing to the other side, never really being able to join the living again.

I was fascinated by this, and I wanted to write a journal that I could publish. Fortunately, I only showed it to one publisher, who was also a friend. She declined. It was too raw, she said. Most illness memoirs should be written with the benefit of hindsight, when there is a distance and understanding of the experience. The nature of my illness, the limited time I had, could mean that I wouldn't have that luxury.

I'm not sure that I wanted to write an illness memoir, exactly.

I just wanted to try and pin down this strange new planet that I had found myself in — the land of the walking dead. Because that is what I did even prior to diagnosis: I documented my life, whether in fiction or in memoir.

But as I look back (admittedly still with not all that much hindsight), I can see it would have been a mistake to publish those pages. In some ways, their rawness is their strength, but the cost of sharing my thoughts of that time could have been too much for me and for the people I love. They may also have been unpalatable for most readers.

Instead, I chose to write a regular column for *The Saturday Paper*. By taking manageable bites out of my experience, and only once a month, I could massage it, shape it, smooth the sharp edges.

Writing the column was a saviour for me. Having to do something (other than just wait around to die) gave me a purpose. It was also my way of saying that I was still me. I could still write.

But eventually, it depressed me. I felt in danger of being defined by my illness, and, above and beyond that, there is always something slightly distasteful in writing about oneself (although I do it a lot). You know you are creating a fiction and this is what you are selling, but because many readers, understandably, don't know the difference between you as you live and you on the page, your writing is often uncomfortably close to prostitution. The line between the story of yourself and your actual self becomes hard to navigate.

Some years ago, I wrote a series of autobiographical essays called *Births Deaths Marriages*, which I found excruciating to publicise. As part of doing the interview rounds, I was asked to read excerpts from the essays on the radio. It was a pre-record, just me and the ABC sound man (whose name I can't remember — I did my best to blank it out) together in a studio. For three days I read to him, careful not to pop my p's or hiss on my s's. I hated the intimacy of it, him thinking that he was privy to all my secrets — although in reality he was probably just listening to the sounds that I was making and not the words, or sense, as such.

On the last day, I read the essay about losing my virginity. I'd been dreading it, steeling myself for it, trying to ignore the bearded man behind the glass who never said a word, other than 'go back to the beginning of that sentence'.

When I finally finished, he looked at me and shook his head.

'Why on earth did you write that one?' he asked.

The shame.

I was swallowed alive by the shame of it.

My column about cancer was easy at first, but at the end of my first six months of treatment, I wanted to give it up. I felt I had nothing left to say, and because I was trying to spin new material out of the same raw ingredients, it felt dishonest. Everything came down to the same pinprick piercing the page: We are all dying. We all should be living life appreciating the beauty of the ordinary. But so often we don't. And this is the eternal human paradox: the only way we can cope with our mortality is to ignore it, to live as though we have all the time in the world.

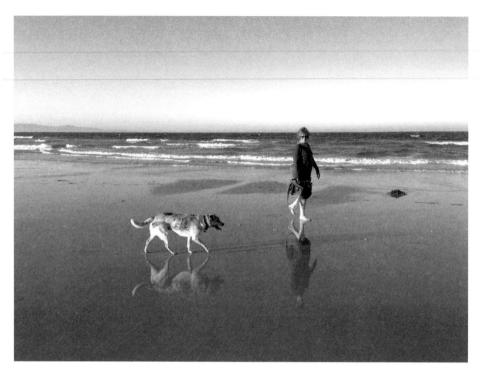

Georgia and her dog, 'Sunday', South Coast NSW, October 2014

I am wary about reducing my daughter, Odessa, to words. She is a fluid, living, breathing creature that I have no right to capture. I don't want to hone my craft on her, and I am aware that every time I mention her, I will avoid getting to the essence of her (and not just because that is always difficult to do with someone you know well).

I *will* tell you that she loves language. It is no surprise. She has been surrounded by people who read and write books. This is the world she has known. She devours books, writes beautifully, and also studies Latin and French (the latter she speaks very well, but more about that in a moment).

Not long after I was diagnosed, Odessa began her final year of high-school studies. She calmed herself by doing Latin translations. It was homework, but it was also a meditative practice, a slow and steady focus on a puzzle that she could solve. She loved telling me the complexities of this work — the way in which the subject could be buried in a piece, and you would have to hunt for it, never able to really make sense of

what goes before until, there, you'd fished it out.

I often asked her how she would say something in Latin. The question didn't make sense to her. The purpose of studying Latin was to translate a piece of text into English. Her brain worked in this groove. She couldn't play the record backwards. And it was the process that mattered more than the end result, like wiping fog from a window so that you could see into another time and culture, a little bit more revealed with each word of the puzzle.

Through her language studies, she has a better grasp on grammar than I've ever had. She was given grammar exercises in English at the beginning of high school, and I was totally ill-equipped to help her with them. Once we got beyond modifying clauses, I would just shrug, helplessly.

When I was schooled, the prevailing wisdom was that it was unnecessary to teach grammar, unless learning a foreign language. French classes were the first time I learnt the names for tenses, and what it was that each tense did. I have never grasped the subjunctive (Odessa tells me it is like a mood). I also frequently trip on the past perfect — how long can you go on for in this convoluted tense, and when is it okay to slip into the simple past?

My grasp of English is like most native speakers. It is as though I am in a house that I know well, with all the lights off. My familiarity means that it is rare that I knock something over or cause an accident, but it would certainly be very difficult for me to explain to a visitor how to find his or her way around each room.

When Odessa had to choose her subjects, both her grandmothers were keen for her to do French.

Andrew and I were not fussed either way.

She chose Latin, and as most people advised her against doing two languages, she also chose textiles, later regretting her decision.

Jhumpa Lahiri, a short-story writer and novelist I have long admired, talks about the necessity of going out of your depth, of swimming too far from the shore, if you really want to learn another language.

Lahiri had been obsessed by Italian for two decades, but it wasn't until she decided to live in Rome and write in Italian only (I wonder how her publishers greeted her news) that she began to gain something akin to fluency.

Odessa decided to take the same approach.

When she was fifteen, she went on an exchange to a small village in Belgium for five months. She lived with a French-speaking family and attended a school some miles from her home.

Before she left, she immersed herself in as many Apps as she could find. 'Coffee Break French' was a particular favourite of mine. With heavy Scottish accents that miraculously morphed when they spoke French, Mark and Anna would converse — running through everyday scenarios like booking a hotel room, or complaining about a meal (what would you do if you discovered a fly in your soup?).

In the last four weeks before Odessa's departure, I took her to one-on-one French classes every Saturday morning. The

teacher was Parisian, she had a lisp, and she spoke rapidly. She was emphatic about the need to understand the foundations of grammar.

Outside the controlled world of the App, Odessa began to realise how little she knew, and she filled notebooks with rules and exceptions, vocabulary and conjugations.

When she arrived in Belgium, she was overwhelmed. Her first Skype calls were excited, but then the reality of how difficult and lonely it was took over. Her host family didn't speak much English and were dismayed at how little French she spoke. However, Odessa is nothing if not determined. She wanted to come away speaking French, if not like a native, then definitely like a Belgian — a joke often used by the French to belittle people who speak their language with a different accent.

She made a pact with the one other exchange student at her school. Despite having to rely on each other for company, neither of them would speak English (Sofia was Brazilian and spoke fluent English and Portuguese). Odessa also shunned radio and television, as so much was in English, and she only read in French.

All crutches were removed. I don't know how she did it.

Our weekly conversations, which thankfully were *not* in French, would often start and end with tears. I remember her talking about her struggle with a 1000-word essay on the definition of philosophy — in French, of course — and the absolute panic she felt at having nothing to say, no way to articulate her thoughts.

I know that the few times I tried to write to her family over there, I found my limited grammar and vocabulary made it very difficult. I had schoolgirl French, most of which I'd retained, but I couldn't bend the words to suit my purpose. I became like a child, unable to convey anything other than the most simple commands or wishes.

Her host mother booked her into lessons for new migrants, and she went each morning before school. She was the youngest in a class full of Eastern Europeans and refugees from Africa and the Middle East. That, too, was a life lesson in itself, one in which she came to see how privileged she was.

At the end of the five months, her progress was remarkable, and she was justifiably proud of her achievements.

Now that she is home, she feels her French deteriorating, despite listening to podcasts and news, and still reading novels in French. Because it's one thing to understand a language, but another to speak or write it, to inhabit it truly. I know she'll go back, but first there's talk of South America and mastering Spanish, which she is keen to do next.

I have an uncle who has lived most of his adult life in Italy (the one whom we went to visit in Rome). He is a native English speaker who speaks Italian fluently. He also speaks French and Spanish almost perfectly. It is curious how his personality changes according to the language he is adopting. We used to laugh about him being a morose English man, but when he talked in Italian he became alive, gesturing with his hands, passionate and capable of holding his own with a Roman in an

argument about a parking space.

When Lahiri abandoned the language in which she wrote, she found herself constrained, and in that constraint was excitement. She was learning to write again, in a different register, without the baggage of her own personal history as a successful writer. Writing in another language is also an opportunity to innovate, to break with stylistic customs and literary traditions.

It is like taking a journey. In an unfamiliar environment, your senses become alert again; you notice the dusty smell, the intense colours, the way in which the light is softer, the cacophony (or absence) of noise. When you return (and for the time being, Lahiri is swearing she will not return), the familiar is delightfully unfamiliar. All that you took for granted is now new, and for a brief time, your senses remain switched on, attuned to that difference.

Beckett is another famous example of a writer who abandoned his native language, choosing to write in French — perhaps to escape the long shadow of Joyce over his own words. Conrad and Nabokov also chose to write in English, despite being Polish and Russian respectively.

There are other ways in which you can impose constraints on your writing, and there were various exercises that I used to do, both for myself and occasionally when I taught. My favourite was writing a story without the letter 'e'. I had to hunt for different words, and I had to distort sentence structures to come up with a cohesive narrative.

My first short story published in an anthology was born

out of this exercise — it was about a fledgling magician who was determined to make his girlfriend disappear.

Georges Perec, the son of Polish Jews who emigrated to Paris, made a career out of writing with constraints. His 300-page novel, *La Disparition*, published in 1969, didn't once use the letter 'e'. Interestingly, as his own name is littered with e's, the novel ensured the author's own disappearance. His novella *Les revenentes* (published in 1972) was a companion piece in which the *only* vowel used was 'e'.

Unlike Lahiri, Beckett, and Nabokov, I have not chosen to write in another language, nor am I willingly writing with constraints, as Perec did. But occasionally, it still feels as though this is what I'm doing.

At first, after the brain surgery, I had to work hard to communicate. The surgeon tried to reassure me that it would get better.

'Most people wouldn't even know that you have an affliction,' he said.

He told me I was like the Roger Federer of English. I had been injured. He wouldn't put me back on the court to play competition tennis, but if I was having a social game, I would still be totally competent.

He also said there was not much point in going to speech pathology.

'What you feel is wrong is too subtle to benefit much from the exercises they would do.'

Since those early days, I have become stronger. I know that.

But I also know that the kind of tumour I have grows back aggressively, and usually in the same place. It is likely that my language will worsen, and when I panic, I send Andrew emails (using every vowel I need) with instructions from the mundane to the more complex: from how to pay Anne's nursing-home fees, to my wishes regarding stopping treatment.

When I was young, Anne and I used to go to fetes and second-hand shops, scouring the white-elephant stalls and shelves for anything by Ethel Turner and Mary Grant Bruce, as well as Angela Brazil. We had a shelf for our collection of books, separate from all the others.

Of these, I liked the Angela Brazil stories the best. Most of them were set in boarding schools, with midnight feasts and hockey or lacrosse matches. But secretly, I liked Enid Blyton's boarding-school books even better. Anne didn't approve, and I had to buy them out of my own pocket money. They weren't nearly as pretty — often dog-eared paperbacks with grubby covers and no illustrations — but the stories were thrilling, and more satisfying than the others. Nevertheless, I kept them separately, away from the special collection that Anne and I had.

My father loved Ethel Turner — particularly *Seven Little Australians*.

Years later, I watched a re-run of the ABC miniseries with Odessa, and I was struck by how cruel the Captain was. He

was a man of brooding silences and an explosive temper, and everyone tiptoed around him.

He was like my own father.

'Turn it off,' Odessa said. 'It's horrible.'

Anne had a Hans Christian Andersen fairytale book from her own childhood, which she donated to our collection. The coloured plates were exquisite — deep blues, greens and crimsons, even gold and silver — and each was faced by a fine page of tissue paper that made them all the more special. My favourite was 'The Nightingale and The Rose', with the thorn piercing the breast of the bird as it sang by the frosted light of the moon.

I also loved *Struwwelpeter*, cautionary tales for children with illustrations both gruesome and fascinating. The two that remained scored on my mind were the story of the thumb-sucker, whose thumbs were cut off by a tailor with giant scissors, and the story of Augustus, who stopped eating his soup for no apparent reason, and wasted away.

When Anne moved to her house by the sea, there was no longer any separation between her books and our collection. They were all in the floor-to-ceiling bookshelves that lined her workroom. The children's books were on the bottom shelf, and some of the more precious ones were in a cupboard whose door was latched.

In the few weeks when we were cleaning up Anne's house for sale, we asked Odessa to tidy the books. She had loved them, frequently sitting on the floor reading them while Anne wrote

or talked on the phone; first, the children's ones, and then, as she got older, she discovered buried treasures: *The Floral World*, *Adventures in Tibet*, a beautiful dictionary of nursery rhymes, and an illustrated edition of *The Canterbury Tales*, to name a few.

The bookshelves had become full a few years ago, but Anne kept buying books, despite her decreasing capacity to read. There were piles in each of the rooms, on every surface. Some were gifts, some were written by friends, but the vast majority of the last purchases were books on the brain: easy exercises to improve brain function, meditation techniques, or works by neurologists. I knew she'd also been subscribing to online exercises for enhanced cognitive function, as well as pills, which she never took, but each time I cancelled one subscription surreptitiously, she filled out another.

Odessa packed the books that she wanted in boxes, and I carted the collection of children's books that Anne and I had amassed to the spare room. There was a bookshelf in there as well — there were bookshelves in most rooms of that house, even the bathroom.

I decorated the room as though it were a child's — a brightly coloured quilt on the bed, a rocking chair, and all the boarding-school books on display. I had never lived in that house, but Odessa had often stayed over in that room, and I know she'd loved her nights there.

I was grieving terribly — for my mother and for myself — but I couldn't let myself cry. I just had to get the house ready for sale. I was in a tunnel, determined not to see anything but

the immediate task at hand.

When I finished the spare room, I went down to check each of the other rooms. It was the last day before the open inspections were due to commence, and I'd asked Andrew and Odessa to give me a moment alone, just to be in that house by myself. They told me they would meet me in the café across the road.

In Anne's workroom, she had a corkboard near the phone. We had taken it down when the house was painted, and it was still bare. I hastily decorated it with a pile of photos in her cupboard.

There were the dogs, Bibi and Clodagh (she's always had a thing for pretentious dog names); her grandchildren (I loved the one of Odessa chasing balloons across Anne's workroom); holidays with her brother in Italy; and her own children — Joshua and me.

I was almost undone by this final task. Andrew drove me home, and I kept my eyes closed, wanting to shut down, wishing that looking back had made me stone, trying to just focus on my breathing, slowly and deeply.

As we pulled up in Marrickville, I finally managed to tell them of decorating the pin-up board.

'I felt as though I was creating a museum of happiness,' I said.

Odessa looked at me, eyes wide, seizing on my words, and I knew what she was doing.

'Don't you dare,' I told her. 'I'm still alive and I thought of it.'

She knew. What a title. The Museum of Happiness.

There was one book that we somehow missed in the sorting. It was Anne's first publication, a story in a girl's anthology. It was accepted in her early twenties. I don't remember its title or what it was about, but she often told me how proud she had been at the time. It was seeing her work in print — not in a newspaper or magazine, but in an actual book.

I, too, remember when I was first published — it was a story about an amateur magician who wanted to make his girlfriend disappear (the one originally inspired by the writing exercise where I made the letter 'e' disappear). After so many rejections, I finally had been published. I was on my way to becoming a writer.

Odessa has just recently had her first short story published in an anthology. Curiously, the fact that it will be in a book with pages still matters to her, even though she is a child of the digital age.

Her story was inspired by one that Anne had told both her and me — when Odessa was a young girl, and when I was a child before her.

In her early teens, Anne had emigrated to Perth from Malaya after the collapse of Singapore. I am ashamed to say that I am very sketchy on the details, partly because Anne's stories changed often (the drama was much more important than the facts), and partly because I was never one for history, the great events. I liked the smaller details: the friendships, the squabbles, the rivalries.

Interestingly, Anne did write about this time in her book,

Waging Peace, but I knew that so much of this work had been affected by Alzheimer's, I couldn't turn to it for any kind of truth.

But what I do know is that there were three women who fled to Perth with their daughters. Those daughters were Anne, Patsy, and Judy, and their fathers weren't with them — at the time of the story they didn't even know if they had made it out of Singapore alive, although Anne's father did eventually make it to Perth, some months later.

Anne was shy and vulnerable. Patsy was a bully.

One day, Patsy made her eat a whole rose: tissue-paper petals, leaves, stalk, and thorns.

'Why didn't you refuse?' I asked, horrified at the thought. How could you swallow a thorn?

She was scared of Patsy. It wasn't that she'd hurt her in the past, but Patsy had a hold on Anne, and she was afraid to say no.

When Anne told the story to Odessa, Odessa also asked the same question.

Just as I had never forgotten this story, Odessa also didn't forget, and she teased it out, strand by strand, like floss, until it was ready to be pinned down, there on the page. Her first published story. I know this process — the painstaking unravelling, like a spider building its web, again and again each time it's removed, until finally it's complete, in all its intricate and magnificent detail.

After the news of Odessa's publication, we went to visit Anne in the nursing home. Sometimes, when I talk of Odessa, she

momentarily surfaces out of the goldfish bowl of Alzheimer's where she spends most of her time, swimming round and round, trapped, bumping up against her own reflection.

So, I came up with a plan. I told Mary and Sarah and Annabel and a few others whose names I've forgotten and whose faces have faded from my memory that we should put her through a test – to see if she really belonged.

The following lunchtime I came to school with one of Mrs Shelly's crimson roses in hand. I walked over to Abigail, who looked up and smiled the shyest, loneliest smile. I sat down next to her, the sun beating down on my back, and told her that I would be her friend if she ate this one crimson rose, thorns and all.

I often think about what would have passed through her mind as she cast aside her dignity. Maybe it was just a simple, desperate longing to belong. I too could relate to that. I... ared – my popularity seemed to be all... ild catch Ma cryin...

...couldn't keep fighting this tide of curiosity.

...ver once made a...

Excerpt from Odessa Blain's story, 'A Southern Rose'

'So what do I do now?' she often asks, and it breaks my heart.

I tried to tell her that Odessa was going to be published, to remind her of the story of the rose that she'd told to Odessa and me, but it didn't penetrate the dense fog.

'Do you remember Patsy?' I asked.

She just looked at me blankly.

I also told Rosie of Odessa's story. This habit was deeply ingrained. Whenever I had news, I would tell Andrew first, Anne and Rosie next.

It was Anne who had originally introduced me to Rosie. They had met through the Australian Society of Authors, where they were on the Committee of Management together.

Anne told me I would love Rosie; she was fierce and warm and honest and intelligent. It was the first time my mother and I had made a mutual friend, although we managed to keep our friendships separate.

I would often joke about how skilfully Rosie walked the tightrope that was the relationship between Anne and me. Whenever we fought — and it became more frequent when the Alzheimer's was first making itself evident, and I was trying to get Anne to face up to it — we would hang up the phone, both of us crying or shouting or both.

And then it was a race to speak to Rosie. When I dialled too late and heard the engaged signal, I knew that Anne had got there first, and it would be an hour or so before I could get my turn.

Rosie listened and advised while never betraying our confidences. We both trusted her.

Since the first months of recovery after her surgery, it had become increasingly hard to speak to Rosie on the telephone, and with neither Anne nor I able to drive, we were usually restricted to this means of communication.

I missed her.

She often managed a few words at the beginning of our conversation, but then she would find it more difficult. I was never sure how to navigate it. I usually just talked, but then

I would become afraid that I was swamping her with words. I know myself that there are times when I can't cope with too much talk. I feel my brain start to short circuit. I have to concentrate intently, and it is tiring.

This time, I called Rosie primarily to tell her that Anne had had a fall and an operation. I wasn't entirely sure whether she took it all in. I wished we could speak face to face, so that I could see the comprehension (or not) in her eyes.

But then, I told her about Odessa.

Her whoop of delight was instantaneous, her words were fluent, and her joy was beautiful.

'How wonderful,' she said. 'How absolutely wonderful.'

Although it took a long time before Anne had the confidence to call herself a 'Writer', before she proudly declared it on her passport — no crossing out of words, just 'Writer', capitalised, in bold letters — prior to that, she had had a long and successful career with words.

She always put her achievements down to the cultural cringe of Australians.

'It was just because I was English,' she said.

This may have been somewhat true, but it wasn't the sole reason.

Sometimes, she attributed her success to my father's success.

Again, I'm sure that helped, but there was another factor: Anne, herself.

She had chutzpah and sass, and she always dared to put herself forward.

She was a media personality before the term was even coined. She had regular spots on commercial TV; she was the first female talkback broadcaster in Australia; she wrote newspaper

columns; she advertised soap powder; and then, in the Whitlam era, she was appointed to the Royal Commission into Human Relationships, a commission that examined social issues such as abortion, age of consent, domestic violence, and homosexuality.

This last role gave her the courage to divorce my father. Later, she told me that as she listened to battered wives around the country giving testimony to the Commission, she realised that she, too, was one.

But it wasn't until she had published *Tell Me I'm Here*, a book that changed the landscape of mental illness, both socially and medically, that she called herself 'Writer'.

This book was her story and the story of my older brother, Jonathan, who had schizophrenia from when he was about twelve years old, or perhaps even earlier. Anne went from doctor to doctor, psychiatrist to psychologist, and from treatment to treatment, trying to keep him alive. So little was known about the illness, and so much shame was attached to it. In the end Jonathan died, overdosing in his early twenties, but her tale, and her love for him, was read all over the world, altering the way in which people saw schizophrenia.

I remember when I read the book in its entirety and I thought: 'She's done it.' It was incredible, it is still incredible, and even now, people come up to me and talk about how Anne's book changed their lives. And every week, without fail, SANE Australia send a bunch of beautiful deep-blue irises to Anne's room in the nursing home.

But Anne — despite being able to call herself a writer by the

very fact that she'd had a book published that had made such an impact — still experienced the niggling sense of not having quite achieved the status she wanted.

She wanted to write fiction. A novel.

She would tell me that I was going to be a 'proper' writer. It was her way of encouraging me, because she knew that this was what I loved doing, but for her there were also definite rungs on the ladder, and she was low, just a step up from journalism, really.

She had the ability to inspire enthusiasm, to make people think they were capable of changing their lives. Recently, when I read Gloria Steinem's memoir about her life on the road, I was struck by the similarities between her and Anne — that optimism, that belief in grass-roots activism, and that capacity to communicate with all people, whether in a piece she had written for publication or in a speech, given to a small group or a huge crowd. If Anne had stayed in England, or perhaps been in America, I'm sure she would have achieved international notoriety.

She was an exciting public speaker. Her eyes widened, she used her hands, her voice was rich, well modulated, she had enthusiasm, and a smile that charmed everyone. She also loved a camera, and I often saw her, tired or harried, transform in front of the lens.

The last public speech I saw Anne give was at a library event where we were both talking about our work. I had just published a short-story collection, and Anne was promoting *Waging Peace*. By then there was no denying that the Alzheimer's was taking its toll.

Normally, I would never have agreed to such a double billing, but I thought it might be good for us to have a weekend away together. I knew she was declining, and I feared trips together would become more and more difficult.

Like so many daughters with their mothers, I always kept Anne at arm's length, wanting a distance from her that she was eager to bridge. I see it now with my own daughter, and I understand it — why she wards me off every time I come in too close. It's a dance of love and guilt, rejection and over-compensation. I swear to myself that I will let Odessa have the space she requires, but I'm sure I traverse this every day.

Anne was thrilled when I rang her up and told her that we'd been invited to speak together, and that I had accepted. We put the dates in our diaries, and, after my initial enthusiasm for the idea, as the weekend approached I began to dread it.

Like so many literary events, it was dismal. A poorly attended lunch in a library where we were expected to join a table (both at separate ones), talk to the other guests, and listen to each other's speeches. I was the pre-quiche entertainment; she was the tea-and-coffee speaker.

I was too earnest, and bored everyone witless. When I came off the podium, I was ushered to a seat where I could sign books if people purchased them. These signing tables are an exercise in humiliation I usually avoid, but there was no escaping this one. No one bought a book, and I was trapped there as Anne gave her speech.

I knew she had become scrambled, but it was awful to

witness how much her brain had deteriorated. There was no order or logic to her words, and she looked so unlike the Anne who loved performing. She didn't know when she should finish. She had no capacity to keep track of time, and I tried to signal to her that she could wind it up. In the end, her words just petered out, and she stepped off the podium, worn and dazed.

The applause was extraordinary, and I was so relieved. The queue to purchase books and have them signed by her was equally extraordinary. Everyone came up to the table, and I sat her next to me, where she proceeded to sign all the copies of my book.

'But I didn't want your book,' people would say to me as she pressed a copy of my short stories into their hands.

I'd never sold so many.

Afterwards, we laughed. I told her I was going to take her with me to each festival, and we'd play that trick again.

But it wasn't long before she became depressed. We met her friends in a coffee shop at the shopping centre across the road from the library. There was a tree in its centre — the whole building had been built around it — and it once would have been magnificent. But recently it had died, leaving bare branches and a few brittle leaves.

We all tried to reassure her, but she knew she had been terrible.

It wasn't that she forgot the words she wanted to use, she just couldn't order her thoughts, and her inability to corral the words into any logical sequence meant her language began to

break down. She had stumbled, speaking like a child shuffling her palm cards, all the numbers mixed up.

I had always been enormously proud of my mother's ability to speak off the cuff, and a little bit in awe of her vocabulary. Even when I was very young, she never used simple words or talked down to me. I remember her describing me as labile (and I was a cry-baby at the time) and I felt embarrassed that I didn't understand what that meant. She used words no one had heard of, words like apolaustic — who describes a man as apolaustic? And when I queried her, she would be appalled that I didn't know the meaning. I always told Odessa that when Anne died, a large part of the English language would die with her.

As I have become older, I, too, have tried to slip certain words back into my everyday conversation, words that are in danger of becoming neglected. If two words come into my head at the same time and one is more arcane, less commonly used, more precise, I reach for that one. Strangely, now that my speech is more impaired, these are often the words that first come to mind; they are my saviours when I feel the gap widen between me and the next word in the chain. I can't grasp the word 'sad' but 'dolorous' is immediately accessible; if I try to describe a sound as sweet, it is 'mellifluous' that I instantly utter.

For a brief time, the Oxford Dictionary had a website dedicated to saving words on the brink of obscurity. You could scroll over them and they would plead with you to adopt them — 'Pick me'. I showed Anne the website once, and there were very few words she didn't know.

Her vocabulary is still impressive, even with Alzheimer's. She also knows the meaning of the words she uses and she can properly weave them into a sentence, but there is now an enormous disjunct between what is going on in her mind and the world as others are seeing it. Her sentences no longer make sense to the people she is talking to.

It wasn't a rapid breakdown, and there is still sometimes a gossamer thread that links her to us.

We haven't been able to get her out of the home for quite some time now, but we used to take her in a wheelchair to a café across the road. It is on the harbour, near a park with shady trees, dogs playing on the shore, and yachts clinking and bobbing, up and down, up and down.

Usually, when we got her there, she would want to go back. We would order a hot chocolate for her, but well before it arrived the agitation would set in. It was too cold, too noisy, her head hurt. The chair was uncomfortable; she needed a cushion. Could the waitress get one for her? She needed one now. It was never more than a fifteen-minute outing, but it was miserable.

Once, on our return, we got stuck in the rain, waiting for the lights, and she was very distressed. We tried to distract her by asking her which boatshed she liked best. The green wooden one? The modern glass one? In the distance, she saw a young man from the Philippines. She was sure that he was the nurse she liked, a man called Russia. It wasn't him, but she kept calling out to him: 'Russia, Russia', becoming increasingly frustrated that he didn't answer.

Sometime later, when she had become confined to the nursing home and we no longer took her out, she told me she went down to the harbour each night.

'I often get lost,' she said. 'I don't know how to find my way back. Last night it was raining, and I saw Russia. He told me he would take care of me, and he led me to a boathouse. It was green, and inside there was a bed. He tucked me up and got in beside me and I slept, both of us there, warm and safe.'

———

If the function of language is to articulate our thoughts, to give access to our inner self, there is no doubt that Anne still has a functional grasp of language. It is just that her thoughts no longer make much sense, most of the time.

However, if the function of language is to give order to our thoughts, to express our inner selves so that others can understand, Anne is losing her language.

Only those who know her, have patience, and have access to her past, both immediate and distant, could decipher the real meaning behind a sentence that she utters. Her childhood in what was then Malaya, her time in England, her marriage, family members, nurses' names, all get thrown into the mix — but most of the time we can disentangle them.

She also still pulls out her old bag of tricks, using flattery to cajole. It is less frequent now, but occasionally I still see her reach for a nurse's hand, look into her eyes, and tell her she is the kindest, wisest person she has met in this place.

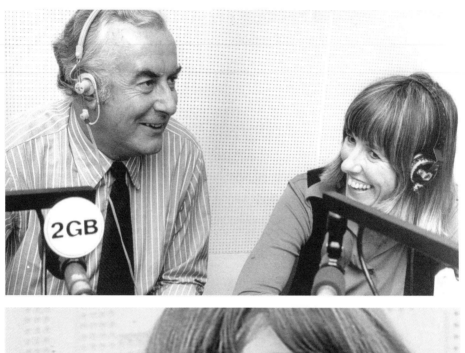

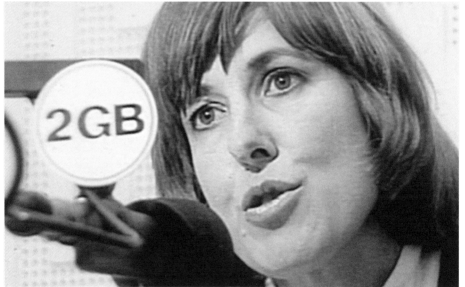

Above: Anne interviewing Gough Whitlam, 2GB studios Sydney, c.1972
Below: Anne Deveson, Australia's first female radio talkback presenter, c. 1970

In terms of reading and writing, skills acquired later than the act of speaking, I don't think she is able to do either.

At first, as her reading deteriorated, it was primarily due to her inability to grasp another's logic, to hold slabs of text in her mind, to remember what went before. Now, I think she would struggle to even say individual words as they are written. In all likelihood, she has forgotten how to perform the actual act of reading.

Once, I held up a word in front of her and asked her if she could read it to me.

She dismissed me peremptorily. 'Of course I can,' she said.

But then she shut her eyes, and I doubt whether she would have been able to make sense of the letters.

Similarly, I don't know whether she could still write words on a page, or type them into a computer. Probably not. Even if she could still form, or recognise, the letters to spell a word, she would have trouble performing the act of writing. It is like her incapacity to dress herself — 'what goes on next?' she asks as she tries to put a sock over her shoe.

When she was first diagnosed, she was determined to write about what was happening to her. She was sure that the computer she had used for writing *Waging Peace* was broken, and she wanted a laptop. By then I had charge of her money. She had lost all grasp of numbers, and I was terrified people would take advantage of her. Thankfully, she soon also lost the ability to purchase online.

To my shame, I resisted at first, trying to hint to her that the

problem was her and not the computer.

She was determined to keep control of her life for as long as possible, and the wear and tear on me was, at times, brutal. I knew she couldn't keep track of medication; she couldn't cook or wash, and she didn't like 'strangers' coming to her house to help her. I lurched from small crisis to small crisis.

Each time she insisted that she was still independent, I wanted to shake her, to tell her that it was only because all of us were there propping up her life.

In retrospect, the truth, as it so often does, lay somewhere in between how each of us were seeing the situation.

I am glad that I eventually relented on the laptop, despite the fact that I don't think she ever used it.

She was desperate to still be herself: a woman who wrote, who translated her experiences into a narrative that so many others could relate to. I now know what she was going through. I did the same thing when I came out of hospital — words, words, words on the page, as though I could somehow build a fortress to encase myself, a word structure so robust that I wouldn't crumble.

I am still doing the same thing.

We never found the laptop when we were packing up her house, but in amongst her stationery cupboard were notebooks filled with new ideas for books, beginnings of short stories, fragments of writing, all done in that year before we put her in a nursing home. Interspersed with them were appointment times, names, instructions, things that she was fearful of forgetting,

her handwriting getting more and more shaky, the lists making less and less sense.

Odessa saved them, tearing out the pages, keeping them, perhaps for some later project, perhaps not.

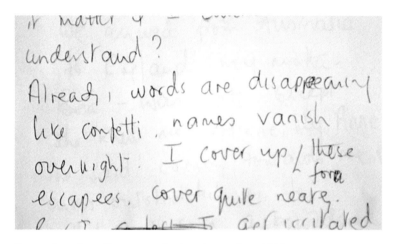

Excerpt from Anne Deveson notebook, written c. June 2014

There have always been a lot of illness memoirs, and, more recently, the 'dying memoir' has been appearing in bookshops. Books by Jenny Diski, Tom Lubbock, and Cory Taylor have all been published since my diagnosis, each charting the progression of his or her cancer and its eventual strangulation of life.

I haven't read Diski's or Taylor's, but I did rapidly skim Tom Lubbock's memoir, knowing that I shouldn't.

Like me, and Rosie, he was diagnosed with a glioblastoma multiforme Stage 4. Like me, he was 51, and the first evidence of his cancer was a seizure.

The tumour was in the language centre of his brain, and he,

too, was a writer: the art critic for the U.K.'s *The Independent*.

He grappled with the loss of his ability to communicate and what it meant to him as a sentient being.

I wasn't strong enough to read it all. I identified too completely — when his seizures started recurring, I thought 'that will be me in x months' time.' When his language worsened, and he struggled to get even a few words to the page towards the end, it was too much. And because I know intimately the fiction of memoir, the need to make sense or shape of the abyss rather than leaving us alone at the edge, I feared the end would be even worse.

I shut the book and put it away.

Language is at the core of our being. The way in which we express ourselves is inextricably linked to who we are and how others see us.

It is also the way in which I have earned my living for a good half of my life.

Unlike my mother, I didn't ascribe to a hierarchy of writing, perhaps because people like her had broken down those rungs, allowing me the freedom to dart from memoir to novel. For me, the line between fiction and life writing is never clear-cut. Each requires drawing on the self and distancing from the self. When Knausgård achieved global literary fame with his epic six-parter, the memoir was elevated even further. This was no longer something that just women did. A man was doing it, and therefore it had to be taken seriously.

I wrote a journal before I started writing fiction, but it was

practice, a fictionalising of the self, a journal written with one eye on the potential audience I was sure I would have. I was trying out styles of writing that were often influenced by what I had just been reading.

In my early twenties, I started getting more serious about short-story writing. I felt both immense pleasure and frustration when I wrote. It was all down to the balance: like a mathematical equation, I had pace on one side of the ledger, and a languid haze on the other; rich and threadbare; dark and light; sparse and intricate — all feeding into each other, a little bit of one, a mass of the other, never forgetting what had gone before, always one eye on the whole and each of its parts. And that doesn't mean equality as such; it means precarious dips, wild races, and then a bask in the sunlight.

Sometimes, I would labour for hours, building clumsy sentence on clumsy sentence, a structure that was squat and ugly and pedestrian, requiring a complete knock-down before I could progress. Other times, I wrote without any awareness of time, and it was so liberating to be free of that constraint.

Once, I said to Odessa that writing was the only activity in which I could forget time, and when you forget time, you forget mortality.

Now, more than ever, it is my lifeline. As I write, I forget I have a terminal illness, even though I am writing about language, knowing that my own is likely to be eroded by the illness that I have. I become so absorbed in the words, every one of them, and the layering, the structure, the balance.

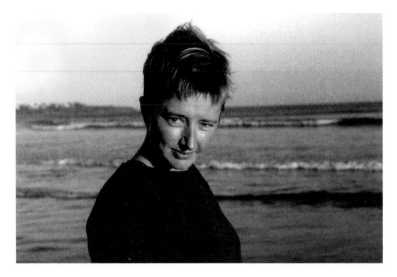

Georgia, Seven Mile Beach, NSW, 1997

When I started writing, it was a long time before I had anything published.

I submitted stories to anthologies and literary journals, and I entered competitions. Anne would tear out entry forms for me, and she would console me when I was rejected yet again.

I am not someone who usually persists in what is seemingly a fruitless endeavour, so it says something about my desire to write that I kept on trying. Perhaps I was also comforted by having read of other writers' rejections. It seemed to be a rite of passage you had to go through.

And through it all I kept reading, learning by osmosis, not yet able to pick a book apart, unstitch it at the seams, but nonetheless gaining a sense of what I liked and didn't like, trying to skirt around the danger of simply emulating a voice I admired.

I eventually decided to apply for a creative writing course at university. I submitted my best stories and dressed up my CV. I was working as a journalist at the time, first at a local paper, and later at a press agency. I wasn't a good journalist — I was too shy and too polite, too eager to be liked to bowl up to someone and ask invasive questions. I also wasn't particularly political. But I could write, always managing to shape a story from not much, and able to do it quickly. I photocopied some of my articles and attached them to my application as well.

Needless to say, I was rejected. Not once, but twice.

I'm not sure what I wanted from a creative writing class other than contact with other writers, both those more experienced than me and those that were on a par with me. I may have also wanted the *chemistry* of a class, the group enthusiasm that can be something more than the sum of its parts.

In terms of learning to become a better writer, I do feel you can teach the elements of writing, and skills to become more adept at navigating your way through a text, tricks to help you keep going when you feel all is hopeless. But there has to be something else, and maybe it is as simple as saying that a writer has to need to write — they have to have a fundamental urge to shape experience through language, to create art out of existence. But where does this need spring from? Your environment? Your genes? A combination of the two?

Most universities offer writing courses now — they're relatively cheap to run and are popular with students, despite the fact the publishing industry is shrinking. And because of

that shrinking industry, many writers have taught at one stage of their career.

Some years after those unsuccessful applications, I taught a short-story course and another one in narrative, at the university to which I'd originally applied.

I was there early on the first day (writers are notoriously punctual), and I was surprised at how nervous I was as my students filed in. I counted down the roll and compared it to the number sitting in front of me. Students whispered in groups of two or three. Some didn't know anyone else in the class, and they were careful to avoid my eye.

At five past one, everyone had arrived. I closed the door.

For one moment my heart thudded, loud and hollow. My palms were sweaty. I remembered reading a memoir written by a teacher who described that first moment in front of a class as one of the loneliest moments she had known.

My voice croaked as I introduced myself, and I looked at all their faces — some eager, some bored already, and some resistant.

Once, I had so wanted to be in their place. Desperately. Now, as their teacher, I questioned what knowledge I could impart. I only had one bag of tricks and I used it for each of the courses I ran, hoping that there would never be an overlap of students doing the two.

Voice. Dialogue. Structure. Point of view. Character.

Each lesson, we talked about one of them. We had examples to discuss. But the students were eager to write, and I was meant

to let them do exercises in the latter half of the class.

Writing in a group was anathema to me. It didn't make sense. Reading your work out before you'd had a chance to digest and edit also seemed wrong. But they desperately wanted feedback. I often wanted to tell my students to go home and just do it — start writing and keep going. Try to figure out solutions for yourself, I wanted to say, and if you're really stuck, come back to class and I could try to advise.

Midway through the semester, we switched to a workshop model. Each student was meant to have a complete draft of their work done, and was asked to circulate it to the others in the class, who would then workshop it for them.

I printed out guidelines for workshopping, and everyone abided by them.

The problem was that providing useful feedback is a skill that has to be learnt. It requires being a reader — as well as a mix of diplomacy, being able to elicit responses from the writer, and astute listening.

Most of my students weren't readers. Every time I mentioned a text to them, some very well known, some current bestsellers, some a little more obscure, they looked at me with blank faces.

Most wanted to be useful, feeling that saying something was better than saying nothing. Most were unable to articulate what it was that they didn't feel worked about a piece, and most couldn't separate personal taste from useful criticism.

There was one student who I thought was particularly talented. She was shy, never said much in class, but always

handed in work that was striking in its strength of voice and originality.

When her short story was workshopped, I was surprised at how lukewarm the rest of the students were. She nodded and didn't say much, but I knew she was close to tears. Afterwards, I took her aside and was completely unprofessional.

'Ignore them all,' I told her. 'Your work is the best in this class. In fact, you are the only one who I think has any chance of being a writer.'

There was another student who was very confident and complained bitterly when I didn't give her a distinction.

'I've always had a D, often an HD,' she said. 'Why did this only get a credit?'

I'd given her feedback when I returned her essay.

I told her to take it home and put it in a drawer. 'Don't take it out for two years. If you still want to know, by then you'll be able to tell for yourself.'

I was glad to give up the work. Like most writers, I wanted simply to write, and not to teach, but like most of the other authors I know, I had to earn a living.

This is an oft-neglected subject in books that encourage being an artist. There is no greater stifler of creativity than obsessing about money. It erodes your time, and it can make you too safe in your art.

Early on, I decided that I didn't want to use the part of me that was essential to my love of writing for anything other

than writing: the daydreaming self, the self that read and could be excited, transported by words. Teaching required me to separate out the ingredients of a written text, as did reviewing, and manuscript assessing — all of which brought me perilously close to dismantling the thing I loved. I wanted to keep the mystery of the whole, because really good writing is always so much greater than the sum of its parts.

But words were the skill that I had, the one thing that I could sell.

Fortunately, a friend of mine gave me a break in copywriting — brochures and websites, annual reports and speeches.

I was surprised at how much I loved it. Again, the mathematics of it appealed, but it was a different kind of balance — a simple equation that had a defined answer. There was a logic and precision to the work, a fine surgical skill, particularly when you were on a word count.

You also needed to be able to quickly determine the tone. Friendly? Formal? Quirky? With speeches in particular, I would have to imagine my words coming out of someone else's mouth, imbued with another's personality. I was told X doesn't do jokes (*thank God*, I thought, *I don't do them either*), or Y never does adjectives; the Chief of Staff or Head of Marketing relaying the main gist of the speech that I needed to prepare, as well as the tone of the message. In this one, the gloves are off. Or, softly, softly, don't mention the war.

I liked it: this careful crafting of words that was more distant from myself than my own writing.

And so I have come to be totally reliant on my ability to communicate, particularly in the written form, for both my living and my joy. As the surgeon said, it is like I am an athlete who is injured, a builder who has a bad back, an actor who often loses her voice.

The first time I took on a job after the tumour was removed, talking was still difficult for me, and so was writing creatively. I was asked to do a corporate newsletter for a large organisation. I didn't think they knew about my tumour, and I debated whether or not to tell them. In the end, I decided not.

I was nervous when I agreed to the job. I wasn't sure if I was capable of ordering information so that it was logical, and flowed — but also so that it was precise.

Apart from being slower than I used to be, it was still there. Strange how my capacity to order information in a written form was still largely intact, unlike my ability to verbally articulate instructions.

I was so relieved that I wept. This part of me was okay. For now.

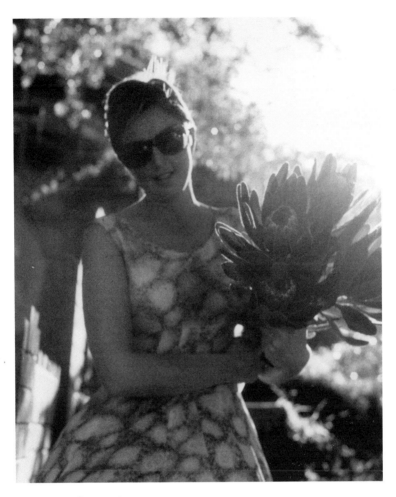

Georgia, Bondi c. 1995

In happy times, my mother used to read poetry to my father. They would sit in his study, each taking a leather armchair, the book of poems open on my mother's lap. He often told us she had a beautiful voice, and it was, rich and smooth — a voice like molten chocolate, an interviewer once said about her.

I recently listened to an audio recording of her made before I was born. I was surprised at how reedy her tone was, how thin and high. She'd had to learn to use her breath, and she often credited my father with helping her.

I can still recall her voice. Sitting next to her as she read to me; talking to her on the phone (we often talked several times a day); listening to her as she conversed with friends. It was a voice that became more confident with age, sun-ripened and warm, until she tilted off into the world of Alzheimer's, the illness infecting every part of her, even her speech, which has become querulous, angry, and confused, although occasionally she reverts to how she was and suddenly issues an imperious command, or a genuinely curious question.

Sometimes, my father would record her poetry recitations on a reel-to-reel, carefully wiping the gleaming silver machine before setting it up in his study. I think she liked reading to him, although I always found it deeply embarrassing. There was something sexual in the act, or perhaps it was simply that in these moments they enjoyed each other's company, and the strangeness of this disturbed me.

He liked it best when she read Edgar Allan Poe, particularly his last complete poem, 'Annabel Lee'. The death of a beautiful woman, whom once dead is safe to worship, would have appealed to my father immensely.

My mother always paused before the last line — 'In her tomb by the sounding sea' — her voice capturing the desolation of setting and soul perfectly.

With his head in his hands, my father would sit, feeling it.

My personal favourite was 'The Raven', who answered all queries with one word: 'Nevermore'.

Again, a beautiful woman, this time called Lenore, had died. Sitting by the embers of the fire, locked in misery, the narrator learns from the raven that he is doomed to never forget his love; nor will they be reunited in heaven.

Although I liked the fact that Annabel Lee was in a tomb by the sea — imagining the sound of those crashing waves appealed enormously — there was no beating the talking raven, even if he had only one word. But what a word: *Nevermore*.

'Nevermore,' I would mutter to myself.

What doom.

'Nevermore.'

Recently, Odessa told me that if it were possible to divorce language from meaning, the most beautiful phrase in the English language is apparently 'cellar door'.

Some say that Poe, who studied the musicality of sound effects carefully, chose the word 'Nevermore' (and presumably the name Lenore) because it had echoes of this phrase with its soothing long 'o' vowel sound. This may be completely unfounded, but there is no doubt that the coupling of these words is pleasing in its rhythm.

I also liked the word 'Nevermore' for its infinite sense of gloom (I am my father's daughter). I didn't think of it as sweet to the ear for its sound alone.

It is such a hard task to divorce language from meaning. As soon as we learn a new word, it is inextricably linked to the way it can be used. But I tried when Odessa told me about the beauty of 'cellar door', willing myself to somehow wipe the images from my mind as I contemplated the phrase, rolling it around like a smooth pebble.

At first I couldn't, but if you repeat a word often enough, it begins to lose sense, becoming just sounds, with a musicality that might be soft and sonorous, discordant and jarring, or perhaps sweet and still.

And the mind can also play with the meaning. A cellar door can be prosaic — a purely functional barrier from one room to the next — or the words can conjure up images of Mediterranean climates, grapes, wine, joy, or perhaps even a

doorway between this world and another.

We have tried to ease Anne's mind through poetry. She doesn't like it.

We have also tried song. Music and earphones hurt her head, she says.

But one time, it worked. A friend of mine came to visit her. She has a beautiful voice, like a pure spring, and I asked her if she would sing.

In the quiet of Anne's overheated room, she went out on a wire, trembling but sure, like a nightingale as she reached for each note of 'Amazing Grace'. Anne used to sing this song when she ran the bath, the sound of the water rushing in, the steam rising, the smell of bath salts, her children in bed.

Lifting her head from the pillow, my mother joined in, her skin like grey tissue paper, her eyes focused on some distant place that we could not see.

There wasn't a dry eye in the room.

From a young age, Odessa used to stay at Anne's house every Wednesday afternoon, and occasionally in the evenings, when Andrew and I would go out.

Anne picked Wednesdays because that was the day she had a personal assistant, out-of-work friends of mine who did Anne's filing, her shopping, and now played with Odessa. It wasn't that Anne didn't want to look after her; she just didn't want to be committed. Any kind of constraint on her personal freedom always made Anne buck, chafing at the bit.

Odessa was an easy child to look after: self-contained, often content to pretend to read, to play with her fuzzy-felts, and to curl up next to the dog, sucking her thumb and staring off into the distance. She could also amuse herself for hours with crawling across the shopfront that was Anne's workroom, making her way from bookcase to desk, to couch and then back again.

Some evenings when we'd been out to dinner, Andrew and I would pick her up, letting ourselves in Anne's orange front door, turning the key in the lock and closing it quietly. They

would both be asleep in the bedrooms upstairs; Anne in her room, Odessa in the one next door, the same room that I decorated to look like a small child's room when we put the house up for sale.

Anne had wooden stairs painted turquoise (she loved bright colours), and Andrew and I would tiptoe up, trying not to wake either of them. But as soon as we entered Odessa's room, her eyes were open — luminous and dark-green, pools of night staring up at us.

We would tell her to shush, it was just us, don't wake Anne, and she would nod, solemn, before commencing … a whole farmyard of animal sounds. First, there was the quack of the duck, then the moo, the oink, the miaow, the woof, the honk honk, the cock-a-doodle-doo, all before we'd even got her out of the cot. Down the stairs it would continue: the neigh, the tweet, the roar, all finishing with a smack of the lips to signal the fish.

Strange that even now so much language starts with the parroting of animal sounds, although animals (other than the dog and the cat) are not much of a feature of our urban lives. I know we used to have picture books, and would ask Odessa to make the sound of the tiger, pig, or goose in the illustration — sounds learned from us rather than the animal itself.

When Odessa came back from Belgium, she told us that dogs say 'qua' rather than woof. In Spanish they 'guf guf', and in Italy they 'bau bau'. Apparently, pigs in Japan 'boo boo' and bees 'boon boon', while the rooster says 'kukeleku' in Dutch

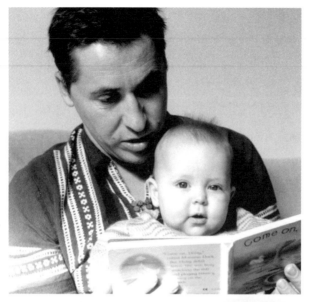

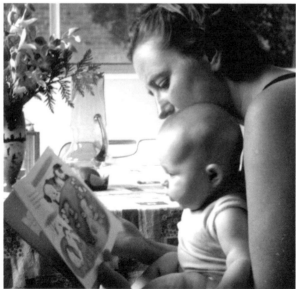

Above: Andrew reading Odessa 'Daisy the Duck'
Below: Georgia reading Odessa 'The Poky Little Puppy'

and 'kukuriku' in Hungarian.

It's extraordinary how we can hear the exact same sound, but make quite different representations depending on the language we speak.

The whole way home, Odessa would continue with her animals, staring out the window, the menagerie less frenetic now, just the occasional trumpet of an elephant or a 'woof woof' from a dog to break the silence. And then when we put her in her cot at home, she would curl up, perhaps miaow, and go straight to sleep, thumb firmly planted in her mouth.

As a child, I often fantasised about animals talking back to us in our language, or about being able to understand them. Many children do. What would animals say? Picture books are filled with examples: from Ant and Bee, to Orlando, the pompous cat.

There is no doubt that domesticated pets have a limited understanding of our words. They can obey commands, often accompanied by hand signals, and anyone who has had a working dog will tell you that there are times when you could swear that they absolutely understand what you are saying.

But as far as getting animals to speak to us in our language — there has been little success. Vicki, the ape, is perhaps the most famous. Adopted by Keith and Catherine Hayes, she was raised as a human baby during the late forties and early fifties. Black-and-white footage shows her dressed in frilly dresses and caps, the Hayes moving her lips for her. She apparently learned to utter 'mama', 'cup', 'papa', and 'up' before she died at the age

of seven of viral meningitis.

Talking requires precise motor skills, involving facial muscles, the tongue, and the larynx (all of which are different in apes), but it also requires a connection to thought. It is an extraordinarily complex system: the way in which we build sentences, let alone whole narratives, to let others know what we are thinking.

Noam Chomsky was the first to posit the theory that our language ability is innate or instinctive. We have an unconscious understanding of language, but we need to be exposed to it early to develop it.

But what happens if we aren't? If a child is raised in silence, could it learn to talk? Is our capacity to learn language a product of nature, nurture, or both?

Scientists call this the Forbidden Experiment. They can't do it themselves, but they seize on any chance to study someone who has been raised without human contact.

A famous recent example is Oxana Malaya, a Ukrainian child who was discovered by authorities in the early nineties, at the age of seven. Initially, it was thought that she had been raised by dogs for her entire life — she could not talk, she barked, ran around on all fours, slept on the floor, and fed herself like an animal. But, as it was later discovered, she had been exposed to language and other forms of human behaviour until she was about three years old. As an adult she has learnt to speak, and does not like being termed a wolf-child.

In 2009, a team of scientists in the United States came up

with a way to conduct this Forbidden Experiment. They took a group of male zebra finches. The males are the songbirds, and the young finches learn to sing by imitating the adult males.

When the young males were locked in cages in isolation, with no adult males to teach them to sing, they only developed a raspy, arrhythmic croak, nothing like the sweet song of birds raised with others in the wild.

Once they had matured, these isolated finches were then released into cages with females. At first, none of the female birds wanted to mate with these strange creatures who could only croak, but desperate times lead to desperate measures.

What was interesting was that the male young of this union imitated their father's inadequate rasp, but modified it with small, systematic variations. By the fourth or fifth generation, birds that were descendants of those who were raised in isolation were singing with all the sweetness of birds that had lived in the wild. This song was already there in the genome of the bird. It just took four or five generations for it to be shaped.

There is another experiment that I love for its whimsy, and lack of cruelty. Professor Simon Kirby at the Centre for Language Evolution at the University of Edinburgh devised a series of made-up words to describe made-up fruits from an alien planet. These words were completely random. So, one fruit could be yellow and diamond shaped, and another could also be yellow, but in round clusters. There would be no common group of letters to signify yellow; in fact, there was absolutely no system to the language at all.

Subject one, let's call her Martha, is taken into a room and shown these brightly coloured pictures of these strange fruits with their nonsense names written underneath them. Martha has a moment to remember them before she is taken into another room and shown the pictures once again, but this time without their names. With no system to the language, Martha inevitably gets most of them wrong. To make any hope of success more dismal, at this stage of the game a few new fruits are introduced. Martha doesn't even notice, and just invents words for the unfamiliar fruits.

The words Martha uses to name the fruits then become the labels affixed to them. Next, Arthur is taken into the room and shown the fruits with Martha's labels. He takes a moment to remember as much as *he* can before being led through to the next room and asked to recall what the names were. Again, he gets most of them wrong, and again, a few new fruits are introduced.

The names that Arthur recalls are then used to label the fruit, and Susan is tested. Susan's names are tested on Matthew, Matthew's for Louise, and so on.

Every time this experiment is conducted, the language used to name these fruits becomes systemised by the time the ninth lot of people are being tested. Each name for each fruit is divided into parts and each has a meaning: one describing the colour, one the number, and one the shape of fruit. These can then be used to name the fruits that have never been seen before.

Kirby's theory was that no one designed language; no one sat down and said it would be useful if it had grammar, clauses and

sentences, verbs and subjects. It is a blind, unconscious process of transmission that will change from generation to generation. It is a living entity, beautiful, fluid, and so remarkable in its adaptability.

But back to Odessa, sleeping in her cot, the curtain lifting and falling in the breeze. She is at home again, after her night-time car ride from Anne's. I'll change the scene a little; she no longer miaows but utters a final 'oo ooo oo', just like Vicki the ape, who should have been left on her own to speak her language with those of her kind.

For humans, these animal sounds are the precursors to talking, often the first sounds that are recognisable, other than ma-ma or da-da. By the time we are five years old, most of us have a vocabulary of 5000 words. An articulate adult has a vocabulary of roughly 10,000 words (I'm sure Anne had about 18,000 at her disposal), and by the time we die, most of us have said about 370 million words in our lifetime, drawing from that far smaller vocabulary.

My half-brother (from my father's first marriage) apparently didn't speak for a couple of years and then, when he finally did, he uttered one fully formed sentence — 'Pass me the hydraulic brake fluid, Dad'.

This is what my father told me, although I find it strange to think that my father was mucking around with hydraulic brake fluid — he was a man who was always immaculate, in seersucker shirts, slacks, a man-bag slung over his shoulder, and a comb in his pocket to tame flyaway hair.

We told Odessa that her first words were uttered after a morning at Nielsen Park. It was a glittering, sparkling Sydney spring day, warm enough for her to get her feet wet in the harbour, build a sand castle, and, when all that was done, eat half a bolognese pie under the shade of a Moreton Bay fig.

As we took her home for her midday nap she uttered her first complete sentences — 'Nice park. Nice pie.'

But they weren't really her first words; they weren't even her first combination of words. Our neighbour at the time reminded me of a prior chant Odessa had used frequently.

As she was trying to stand up on her own, failing every time, she would say 'up down' over and over again, the words running into each other as the time between lurching up and collapsing onto her bottom was infinitesimal. 'Updown, updown,' the call would come as soon as she woke from her nap, a happy sing-song accompanied by the thud of her legs giving way one more time.

Although she didn't say much in that first year and a half of her life, like most toddlers she understood a lot more than she could speak. With only a few words to her articulated vocabulary, I could often give her complex instructions that she could follow.

'Get your jumper,' I would say, and she would go to her room.

'No, not the green one, the yellow one, it's a bit cooler,' and off she would go again, returning with the right jumper.

I found the acquisition of language one of the most joyous times in Odessa's early life. The great leaps she took never ceased to amaze me.

Prior to this, I had found motherhood difficult. I wasn't prepared for the complete dependency of a baby, and, like my mother, I was never very good at being tied down, committed. In those early months, I was often depressed by how little freedom I had. I'm wary about saying that Odessa's increasing vocabulary made her easier for me to mother, because this fast-paced addition of words came at the same time as she began to sleep well and gain more independence. But there was no doubt that our ability to communicate was a large factor in the happiness I began to discover in being her mother.

And it was not just words. Even in the early stages, when her vocabulary was very limited, I could make myself understood and she, too, could make herself understood. Exclamations of delight made my whole being shiny and new: clapping her hands, gurgling contentedly, her soft smile — all were part of the love that kept growing.

There is one phrase that I remember with particular delight, and it always takes me right back to when she was two, with a shock of white-blonde hair, creamy skin, sturdy legs, and a quiet yearning that has always been part of her nature.

She uttered it every time we put her in the backseat of the car to take her to a park. Looking up at Andrew or me as we buckled her in, she would take her thumb out of her mouth and say: 'I hope so the blowflowers.'

It was the dandelions that she was wishing for; cheeks filled with air, and then one, two, three puffs as she sent each silver strand scattering, leaving just a stalk.

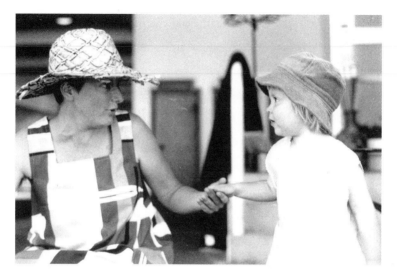

Georgia and Odessa, Bondi, c. 2001

Since my brain tumour was diagnosed, I have become acutely conscious of the passing of time, or perhaps it's more accurate to say that I'm finely attuned to the changing of the seasons.

We moved into this house, with its overgrown garden, a year before I knew I had cancer. Andrew and I ripped out weeds, felled sickly nectarines and plums, and planted: a jewelled bottlebrush, delicate grevilleas, a lemon myrtle, and even a Chinese silk tree. The more mature trees we left along the fence line: a gum, two ashes, and the jacaranda and Illawarra flame trees.

I did not know then that this was the house I would die in.

It was summer and then autumn in the first frenzy of the illness. I watched saplings wither away in the heat, while others grew strong and hardy. When winter came, the brick fence on the western side fell down and the ash lost all its leaves, the

jacaranda and the Illawarra flame tree soon following suit. Curled-up fronds littered the dying lawn, and the garden became winter-bare, the ground traced with wheat-coloured grass runners, stark branches against the impossibly blue sky.

I know that I dread the first appearance of the blossoms, lilac and coral-red, on trees that have been planted side by side to make a spectacular springtime show. My seizure, which had no warning other than the niggling sense that something was wrong with my words, left me collapsed on that carpet of flowers. When the magnificence of that display appears again, I will have had one year out of my expected (if I'm lucky) two.

It is not just the seasons that mark the passing of time in this new world in which I am living. There are scans, constant scans, to track the progression of my illness.

Every three months, I go into the hospital for an MRI, and each time the scans show new nodules or enhancements. They tell me that this could be signs of the tumour reforming, or perhaps just fallout from the surgery or treatment itself.

I regularly buckle under the weight of the uncertainty.

The oncologist is a kind man, in his mid- to late-sixties, softly spoken and always patient with our endless questions. He makes no bones about the fact that he is a man of science; for him, everything is statistics. And there are endless statistics in cancer land.

He is always careful with his words, answering our queries about trying acupuncture or cannabis oil by saying that it would do no harm, but as far as he is aware, there is no evidence to prove

its benefits. Occasionally, he will utter the words 'anecdotally' or even 'hunch', but only when I am looking particularly bleak and he is trying to boost my spirits.

Once again, in his clinic, he called the scan up.

He asked me how I had coped with the last round of chemotherapy.

I told him that I was tempted to lie to him, to say that I had terrible side effects, because I didn't want to go on it again.

He smiled.

There was my brain, multiple pictures of it in black-and-white, and once again there was a new area of enhancement — a silver lining of the cavity where the tumour was removed. It was like a smear, a swipe of frost around the shrinking hole in my brain that once contained cancer, and may still contain cancer.

The MRI report hedged its bets. It might be tumour. It might be dead cells from the surgery and treatment.

'We simply don't know,' he said.

Once again, he booked me in for a follow-up PET scan. These are not as accurate in giving an indication of the size of the potential tumour; instead, they measure the activity. If it lights up like a Christmas tree, it's most likely cancer; if it remains dull, probably not.

Last time, the PET gave us no new information about the nodules. It was equivocal, right on the line, the oncologist said.

'We'll just have to wait and see,' he told me.

Now, the nodules appear to have shrunk, but there is this line, glowing ghostly white, on the MRI.

If it is more tumour, the decision to do more chemo is up to me.

'If the chemo was going to cure you, I would strongly advise you to do it,' he said. 'But with a tumour such as yours, it is not a cure, and we only want to keep you alive if your quality of life is good.'

I know the prognosis, but I try and fool myself that I will be different; I will be the statistical outlier. When I heard his words, my hope sank again, leaden, right to the bottom of the ocean. I had felt strong and optimistic when I had walked into his clinic, but I walked out bowed down by the illness and by the knowledge that I will be ill until the day I die.

The mental battle is extraordinary.

I do well for weeks at a time, and then I come undone. I am on the brink of an abyss so dark and deep I cannot breathe, my head dizzy as I peer down, my legs unsteady, my body ready to topple over the edge.

There is nothing anyone can say to haul me away. I have to do it myself, crawling back from the lip of the crater towards all that I love in life, while knowing that I have to loosen the grip of everything I hold most dear. I am not afraid of dying. What I am afraid of is saying goodbye.

Time and time again, writing is my lifeline, the rope that I use, inch by inch, word by word. It is the way in which I forget myself, even though I am writing about myself. Some days, I feel it is the means by which I am keeping myself alive, escaping the death sentence of this illness for another day.

I am reminded of the story of the King who found out his wife had been unfaithful to him. He decided to marry a new virgin each morning, beheading her the following dawn so that she would have no opportunity to ever cheat on him.

But then he met Scheherazade.

Hidden by her parents, who had wanted to protect her from marriage to this murderous tyrant, Scheherazade had a plan, and she managed to persuade her father to let her marry the King.

On her wedding night, she instructed her younger sister to come to their marriage bed and to beg her to tell one of her many wondrous tales. Scheherazade was a captivating storyteller, and right as day was breaking she stopped, her story on the edge of a knife, telling the King and her sister that she would continue tomorrow night if the King would let her live.

Over one thousand and one nights, she told her tales. During that time, she gave birth to three sons fathered by the King, casting a spell on him with her wit, charm, and beauty. He fell in love with her, and never again threatened to kill her. I hope she also fell in love with him, although it would be hard to love a king with so much blood on his hands — but I'll pretend that she did, and that they had the fairytale ending she deserved.

I'm not laying claim to being as wonderful a storyteller as Scheherazade, but sitting at this desk writing, I feel that there is an inextricable link between my capacity to put words on the page and my being alive. So long as I can keep spinning these tales, I will be spared; I will live to see another day.

I do not know whether I would have become a writer without meeting Rosie. I would have kept writing, I'm sure of that, but I may never have had a book published. Her influence on me is unquantifiable. She is an integral part of who I have become.

I met Rosie when I was in my late twenties.

I had broken up with my boyfriend, with whom I had lived for the last five years. We'd decided to end our relationship after that forgotten trip to Rome, where we had argued over whether a neckline was round or square.

The two of us had lived in a flat with wooden floors and a wooden ceiling painted white. The building was honey-coloured, and every room overlooked the ocean, their window frames a bright cobalt. I never put curtains up, wanting to see the dawn: sometimes rosy pink, sometimes gold, and sometimes like a bruise tinged with mauve. I would wake for just a minute or two, appreciate the beauty, and go straight back to sleep, as you can only do when you are in your twenties and have been out until all hours the night before.

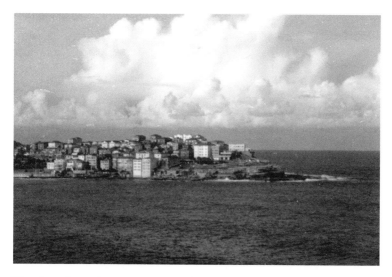

View from Georgia's writing room and flat in South Bondi, c. 1992

After that trip to Rome, my boyfriend and I stayed together for a few months. The end, when it came, was messy. I let him have everything, determined to be rid of him. But I clung onto those rooms overlooking the sea.

This was the flat where I had written my story about the magician who wanted to make his girlfriend disappear, although it was some years before it was accepted for publication. This was my home during the period in which I had countless short stories rejected, and put in my two unsuccessful applications for creative writing courses.

I loved that place, perhaps more than anywhere I have ever lived. Sometimes, in my dreams, I go back there, and it is just as it was. I am at peace again, looking out on the ocean, morning glory tumbling down the cliffs, and then often, in the dream,

the tide starts lapping in through the windows, gently receding and flowing, like a living creature.

In the year or so when I remained in the flat, living with friends, I knew that I needed to change my life. All I wanted was to write. That desire was like a force, threatening to erupt into every given space, no longer capable of being stoppered, and I had to give it more room.

I was working as a lawyer at the time, and I was not good at it. I'd always known that it was the wrong career for me, from the moment I had my first tort lecture and we studied the famous case about the snail in the ginger-beer bottle. I wasn't interested in the company's liability for causing a woman to get sick when she drank the toxic brew. I was far more interested in trying to imagine the woman who had poured herself a glass of that ginger beer (apparently over ice-cream and pears). What was she wearing? Was it a treat? Who was she with?

It seemed to me that there were so many stories buried in the cases we studied, all under a pile of dead language. All that *material*.

I did the minimum I could do to pass, found myself a job, and cried copious tears at the end of my first day. My main task was translating copyright law into plain English, so that artists and other creators could understand it. I wanted to be the artist. Not the lawyer. But I was a good girl. I always did the responsible thing.

Breaking up with my boyfriend freed me from this. I needed to know that something had changed other than him

no longer being in my life. I asked my boss if I could go part-time. At the same time, the lease on the flat was terminated and I moved house. Again I cried, as I carted all my possessions up the hill (no wonder my mother had called me labile), and moved away from the beach to a room that was dark, but had a small sunroom with a mango tree outside.

This was where I was going to write. And I set my computer up on my desk, looking out on to the garden, and I began. Word after word, page after page, until I had eventually created a whole that was an unruly, tangled, awful mess.

It was Anne who suggested that I apply for a mentorship with the Australian Society of Authors. She urged me to ask for Rosie, whom I hadn't yet met.

'You'll love her,' she said.

I wasn't so keen. I had been rejected too often. But in the end, I decided to fill out the application form.

I don't remember what was on it, other than a requirement to submit a few pages of my manuscript in progress. I am also sure that a large part of my success was down to nepotism — Anne and Rosie were in the first throes of friendship, and my mother was never shy about putting her daughter forward. It was embarrassing at the time; now, I love her for it. But like so much that occurs in mother–daughter relationships, I have never told her how appreciative I was.

It was about a month before I found out I was successful. It wasn't like I'd been offered a publishing contract — but the mere fact that I'd won *something* for my writing gave me a boost.

Rosie rang me soon after the news came. She congratulated me on my work and suggested meeting once a month over the next six months. She also said that she didn't want to read my manuscript as I progressed, she just wanted to talk.

I was disappointed.

Secretly, I'd wanted her to be like a de facto editor, marking up my pages and complimenting me profusely, then paving the way for a relationship with an agent, and, ultimately, a publishing deal.

I read two of her books prior to our first meeting. I particularly remember *Lives on Fire* — it was languid, lush, trapped in a tropical torpor, a romantic, almost overheated book. Just recently I read this work again, and without our impending student–teacher relationship to influence my reading, and freed from fashion as works eventually become, the richness of the prose sang to me. She was a beautiful writer, a writer who loved language.

On the morning of our first meeting, I was both nervous and excited. Although I had my mother as a role model — she was also a woman who earned a living from words — the fact that she'd always downplayed herself and her achievements had seeped into the way I viewed her. I was going to meet a genuine author, someone who'd published novels.

When a friend has become so familiar and dear to you, it's hard to remember that person as though she is new again. I want to take myself back there, to the streets of Glebe, to seeing Rosie as I saw her that first morning. It means that I also

have to visualise myself as I was then: on the brink of turning 30, not yet a writer, not yet living with Andrew, nor a mother. The Georgia of that time had so much in front of her, so much life to live, so much happiness to hold.

It's rare that someone is more punctual than me, but Rosie was at the café before I was. She would have been wearing a T-shirt, and a loose skirt, or perhaps a dress, sheer, with flowers on it (she never cared much for clothes, and often wore her favourite items until they were threadbare). My mother never liked that; she could be a terrible snob about matters such as dress, although as she used to get around in sloppy, faded black pants and Indian caftans, she didn't really have any right to judge.

I saw Rosie by the window. She was reading the paper, my manuscript at her side, a glass of hot water in front of her.

She must have been in her late forties then, just a couple of years younger than I am now. As we both chatted, eager to like each other, she told me she lived just around the corner. She loved Glebe — the sandstone cuttings overgrown with monstera and strangler figs, the bohemian community, the cafés, Gleebooks. She had two daughters, who were frequently away on adventures, and a husband she always said she was madly in love with (Rosie was passionate, romantic, enthusiastic, and, like Anne, much more prone to being ruled by her heart than I have ever been).

I know I'm falling into the trap of telling you about Rosie, rather than showing her to you. If I were teaching students, and I wanted them to bring a character to life, I would ask them

to take her to a fictional supermarket and see what she does in there. *An ordinary situation*, I would say to the class. *You could have her cleaning her house, or on a bus. But let's take her shopping.*

My good student, the one that never said much, would whisper quietly that Rosie would never go into a supermarket.

'She lives in Glebe — she'd go to a fruit and veg shop, something much smaller. Or a market.'

Would she do a big shop or buy what she needed on the day?

Halfway between the two, a boy in the back would say, and right at the end she'd sneak a pack of cigarettes in, counting out her change. 'She doesn't really like to admit that she's a smoker.'

She's probably got a deal with the man in the greengrocer, who sells her individual cigarettes, someone else would say.

Good, I'd reply. Now what would she buy?

'She's from New Zealand,' someone would laugh. 'Eggs, sausages, unsliced white bread, and a bunch of irises.'

Would she interact with other people?

Without a doubt — from the shopkeeper, whom she would know, to buying food for others if they didn't have enough money, to chatting to the homeless man with his dog, who was always crouched in the thin strip of shade on the pavement outside.

On that hot, sticky morning (Rosie loved Sydney summers), as Rosie told me about herself, I immediately relaxed with her. I even opened up, more so than usual. She had the gift of making people feel at ease. Over the years of our friendship, I realised that this initial impression hadn't lied, but there was, as there always is, so much more to a person than they initially

show to another. Rosie had passion, but there was also intellect. There was a wicked and sharp sense of humour. And, despite her apparent openness, she was an immensely private person, never revealing her sorrows and disappointments lightly, preferring instead to retreat.

Her love of writing was honed by her intellect. She read widely and astutely, capable of dismissing a book with a few words. The worst sin for her in literature, and in life, was dishonesty. Integrity was the key.

She was also determined not to compromise her life as a writer.

She didn't need much, she always told me, and this was true — she really didn't. She was much less materialistic than I was, and hence didn't get distracted by want (a new couch that could be paid for with just one more job).

She was also much more political than me. When she wasn't writing, she always had a cause that she would throw herself into with dedication and commitment, often working too hard.

But in the afternoons, she was fond of a long bath. Often I'd ring and she'd be in the tub. We'd talk for hours (I have never been one for lengthy conversations on the phone, but she could ensnare me like no other).

She also had a love of hot chips, chicken burgers, and chocolate mud cakes. I rarely ordered food like that (my mother's disdain for fast food has passed on to me), but when our meals came, I often looked at hers with envy, soon helping myself to her plate.

Her circle of friends was extraordinary — from the then Governor General to a girl she met on a bus who'd needed a room for the night. I remember her husband describing her as someone who was always herself no matter who she was with. And he was right. It is a great gift to live like that.

You could still smoke in cafés then, and we both lit up (I had the pack), each relieved that the other was a smoker, although we both considered ourselves social smokers only.

'You're a writer,' she said, as she picked up my manuscript and gave it back to me.

Rosie was apt to make declarations like that. She believed someone was either an artist or they were not (although if they disappointed her, she was quite capable of changing her mind).

I was thrilled, and no doubt I would have blushed.

I don't think it would have been my work that would have led to Rosie's words; more likely, it was that Anne had told her how much I wanted to write, how much I did write. And because Rosie loved Anne, she would have believed in me, and the fact that I was actually doing it, rather than just talking about it, no doubt helped.

She then proceeded to ask me questions — about myself, about what I read, about the books I'd loved and didn't like, and I probably would have tried to impress her with my responses, trying to frame myself as a serious writer. Gradually, the questions focused down to my work, and they were quite broad at that first meeting — what had sparked the idea, what had I struggled with, what did I feel had worked?

If I give the impression that she was airy, she wasn't. She approached being my mentor with the utmost professionalism, including keeping an eye on the time and wrapping up the conversation when our allotted hour was up.

We walked out together, and I asked her about her own writing — was she working on anything?

She was, but she never liked saying. She kept it very private.

I was the same, I said. I never liked talking about my work like this. It was hard for me to do.

She understood.

Over the course of that six months, we met every four weeks or so, and just as she said, she never read my work in between meetings. She interrogated me, fixing her eyes on me, forcing me to answer honestly, to try to articulate whatever it was that I didn't feel was working in the manuscript. Rosie demanded truth. We both demanded that of ourselves, and I love her for that — for the seriousness with which she took my work and me.

We also began to talk more and more about our lives, often stopping by my parked car as I was leaving, extending our meeting for half an hour more with chat and stories and perhaps one last cigarette.

On our second-last meeting, she told me that she'd like to read what I'd written, and a couple of weeks later I dropped it off at her place. It was a draft that I had stripped back and told in the first person. I was excited and nervous and antsy as I waited for her call.

When it came, only a day or so later (because Rosie would

have known how eager I was for her feedback), she laughed that wonderful, rolling laugh and told me that I'd done it.

'My god, girl,' she said, 'what a transformation.'

And with those words, I was away. I was a writer. I had become what I'd wanted to be since even before that afternoon in my brother's bedroom, many years ago, when I first declared that I could read.

I like to look back on that moment of pure joy, because the life of a writer is, more often than not, one of self-doubt. No matter how many books or articles or short stories we write, there are many times when we lose all faith and feel that we are not writers at all. The shell of the self is so easily cracked, and then patched, and then cracked again.

But on that afternoon, I wanted to whoop with delight, just as Rosie did when I told her about Odessa's publication. All the rest — the submissions and rejections; the final acceptance of my manuscript — all of that was to come, but that instant was one of pure sweetness.

In those early days, Rosie gave me some sage advice:

- You've only got so many goes at polishing a manuscript before it loses its edge. It's like polishing a diamond. Never waste one of them.
- Never read over your work when you're tired, likely to be interrupted, or depressed.
- Always interrogate yourself. You know when you're being dishonest.

- Don't dilute the work by talking about it too much.
- Never show your work to a publisher or agent until you feel that it is as good as it can be.

Rosie is no longer my teacher. She is my friend now — one of my dearest friends — but I still live by these words of advice.

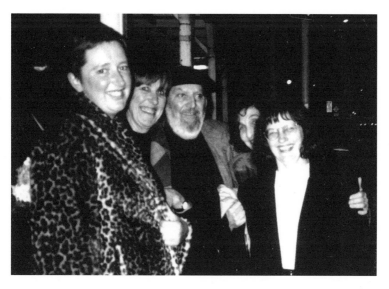

(L-R) Georgia, Anne, Alex and Vivienne Kondas, and Rosie Scott, June 1998 (Georgia six months pregnant with Odessa)

Anne's house was sold before auction to a journalist called Anne. Even though I just wanted it sold, I was pleased by the synchronicity.

All the neighbours were thrilled. The corner shop was just four doors down from her house — Anne had done all her shopping there for years. They told me how much they would miss her. As did the café over the road, at which she'd eaten the vast majority of her meals, the owners often carrying them over for her when she became too ill to leave the house.

'But it's good that we'll have another Anne,' they all said. 'It feels right.'

The new Anne told us that she had always admired my mother.

As soon as she saw the house, she knew it was perfect. She had just accepted a redundancy from her newspaper job and she was going to write a book in the shopfront. She wanted to keep my mother's desk — an old cedar table that Anne had had for as long as I could remember.

Before settlement, we had four weeks to empty the house. The clean-up for sale had involved a lot of tossing, but there was also a lot of stashing — in cupboards, wardrobes, trunks, under beds, and in Anne's shed.

My brother Josh came down from Queensland to take charge of this final stage. In the last year of living in her house, Anne used to talk about what she wanted her friends to have: particular paintings, furniture, a teapot. It was like a game and it soothed her, but each time I asked her to write it down, she baulked. She didn't want to do it, no, not now.

In the end, once we had divided up her possessions between Joshua and me, the grandchildren, and people who were close to her, there was not much left — apart from the books.

And there were so many of them.

Odessa had taken some, we had put others out on the street for passers-by to help themselves to, Andrew had a few — but there were at least four or five thousand left in those floor-to-ceiling shelves that lined her workroom.

No one wants books now. Charities and second-hand dealers say no, even people who sell rare books (and Anne had a few) weren't keen on coming round and looking through her shelves.

Fortunately, the new Anne wanted to take about a quarter.

The rest were packed up in boxes to be 'donated to charity' by the estate dealers whom we had hired to help us with the task. I'm sure they all ended up in landfill.

Most of them were novels, and Anne and I had similar tastes, which meant that I already had many of the books she had.

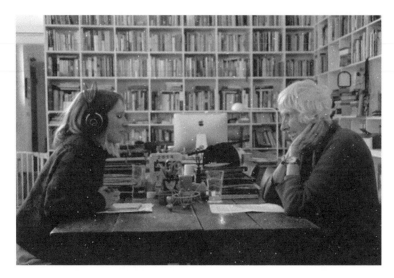

Archivist and filmmaker, Sari Braithwaite, with Anne in her workroom, June 2014

When I first started writing, I used to think that fiction was outside the confines of fashion, but, like all art, there are styles that go in and out of vogue, and most books, no matter how successful they are at the time, are eventually forgotten. I look at my own bookshelves and can see the various stages of my life, like sediment. Every few months or so, I do a sweep of those shelves, giving some to friends, some going straight to the recycling.

These days when I buy a new book, it is rare that I keep it. Usually, I just read it and pass it on. This is partly a product of my acute awareness of my mortality, but prior to the news of my tumour, I had started to toss books anyway — something that I would have found inconceivable in my youth.

Sometimes, I wake in the middle of the night and remember

a book that Anne had owned, and wonder whether Josh, or the new Anne, or any of her friends saved it. Like the anthology that her first story appeared in, or the early Tasmanian book that she once told me was very valuable.

'It's worth about $150,000,' she said at the time.

It was about eight years ago. We'd been to a movie and were out to dinner.

I spluttered on my soup.

I'd had no idea that she had a book worth that much. It's strange how value attaches itself to the object, distinct from the beauty or wisdom — or lack of — contained in the words or illustrations. This value is to do with rarity, condition, age, perhaps an error in a particular print run, and, of course, whether anyone is willing to pay the asking price.

'Why on earth don't you sell it?' I asked.

She told me she was happy to sell it, she just didn't have time to chase up dealers.

I offered to help.

She was delighted. 'You can take half,' she said. 'As commission.'

At the time, I was completely broke. We'd just bought our first house in Marrickville (the one prior to the one we are in now) and had a hefty mortgage. The house had only a hose for a shower and an outside toilet. I'd do the bathroom, I thought, and pay off a chunk of what we owed.

'Are you sure it's worth that much?' I wanted to double check. Numbers were never her strong point.

'That's what I was told,' she said.

'Who by?'

'A book dealer quite some time ago.'

I was so excited that I drove over to her house before nine the next morning.

She was always up early, sitting at her computer, or perhaps making phone calls, and she was delighted to see me again so soon after our date the previous evening.

I had to remind her that I'd come to sell the book, the one that she'd told me about, the $150,000 one. Remember?

She didn't at first, and then she did. 'The Tasmanian one?' Even before the Alzheimer's, she was frustratingly vague.

She looked over the shelves, searching through the older books, most of which were together, taking out a few — 'no, that's not it' — until she put her hand on one with a red binding: 'There it is.'

She leafed through the pages. They were spotted with age. 'We might have to get it repaired. We should probably get some advice. Apparently, it's worth about $1500.'

I looked at her. 'It's worth what?'

She repeated herself.

Silly, silly me. I should have known. Zeroes had little meaning for her. I looked at her, absolutely devastated. All night I'd been fantasising about my newfound wealth, and now it had shrunk to $750, if I was lucky.

I put it back in the shelf and told her that I'd investigate. 'Soon,' I promised.

I have no idea what the book was worth — perhaps $150, or maybe $150,000 — but I let it go, forgetting about it once we'd had our coffee, occasionally remembering it, thinking that I should chase up its true value just in case Anne had been right in her initial estimation. Like most of her books, it has gone, but I like to think that it is perhaps in a cardboard box in the back of a second-hand bookshop (not in landfill), awaiting discovery by someone with a keen and accurate eye for its true worth.

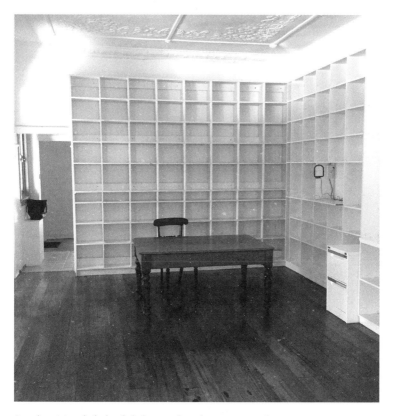

Anne's writing desk, bookshelves, and workroom emptied in preparation for house sale, March 2016

Individual words, too, have a value. Brand names can be worth a fortune, and people will go to great lengths to protect them. Clothing, cars, dishwashing liquid — there is not often much between the items themselves, but the association that the brand name conjures up can be very seductive to the consumer, hence its worth.

Drug companies also have a huge amount invested in brand names like Panadol, and all its derivatives.

I have always called my chemotherapy drug by its generic name — perhaps because my oncologist calls it by that name — and never by its brand name. This is probably part of the reason why it took me so long to learn to pronounce it.

Temozolomide.

Andrew would correct me. 'The first part rhymes with chemo,' he'd say. 'Tee-mo-zol-o-mide.'

But part of my forgetfulness was simply not wanting to remember. I took on a form of helplessness when I was in the hospital system, a feeble attempt at denying that I was ill. For

a few months, I not only refused to remember the name of the drugs that I was taking, but I also didn't remember the floor on which I saw my oncologist, where I had my MRI scans, or where the PET scans were done. Gradually, as the shock began to subside, I became more capable, but I am always surprised at how readily bad news will slip me back into my former feeble state.

Temozolomide, as I mentioned, is the generic name for the drug used in treating brain cancer. Drugs also have a chemical name (in the case of temozolomide this is 3,4-dihydro-3-methyl-4-oxoimidazo[5,1-d]-as-tetrazine-8-carboxamide — a name that I would have no hope of remembering) and a brand name. The brand name is Temodal in Australia, Temodar in the United States.

Naming drugs is big business. When a drug is first discovered it's given its chemical name, which describes its atomic or molecular structure. Because this name is so cumbersome, a shorthand version is developed so that researchers can easily reference it.

When a drug has been approved by the relevant government agency for ensuring that it is safe and effective, it is given its generic and brand names.

Drug makers propose generic names around their compound's chemical make-up. According to my oncologist, there's an art in this. The name's stem describes the structure and function of the drug, and the company can then tack on syllables of their choice. Generic and brand names must be unique to prevent them from being mistaken for another drug when it is prescribed, or when a prescription is dispensed.

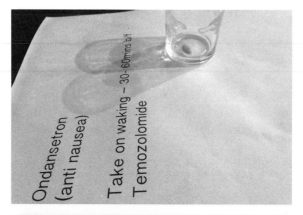

Ondansetron (anti nausea)

Take on waking – 30–60mns b/f

Temozolomide

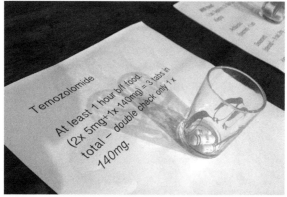

Temozolomide

At least 1 hour b/f food. (2x 5mg+1x 140mg) = 3 tabs in total – double check only 1 x 140mg.

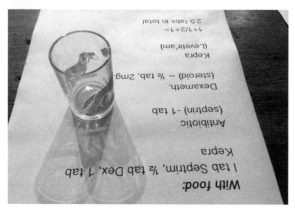

With food:
1 tab Septrim, ½ tab Dex, 1 tab Kepra

Antibiotic (septrin) - 1 tab

Dexameth. (steroid) – ½ tab, 2mg.

Kepra (Levetir'am)

1+1/2+1= 2.5 tabs in total

Georgia's daily morning chemotherapy medications

125

However, the drug company also wants the generic name to be unpronounceable, impossible to remember. This is because there is a small window when the drug is under patent and it can be marketed under its brand name. What you want is for doctors to remember your brand name when the drug is no longer under patent and everyone is free to market it. No one knows what sildenafil citrate is, but everyone knows what Viagra is. Brand names are catchy, often related to the drug's intended use, and relatively easy to remember. But they are also nonsense words — worth a fortune to the company that markets the drug. My favourite brand name of one of the many drugs I take is Ondansetron — an anti-nausea wafer I swallow before my chemo. There's something of a chemical dance-party ring to its name, almost steampunk.

After an initial thirty days of radiation treatment, which followed the surgery, I have been doing chemotherapy alone. Ever since this time, I have been living under the shadow of possibly extending the time I am on temozolomide, or perhaps trying another chemotherapy drug, or even other treatments, one of which is completely unpronounceable — bevacizumab. Even Andrew gives up on this one and calls it Beelzebub, much to the oncologist's mirth.

Recently, I was given a brief break from the treatment.

For the first time, my scans appeared to be clear. I almost kissed each of the doctors in my joy as they told me the news. They didn't want to see me for another three months.

Three months, I thought. *Three months.*

I have to do so much living.

It was the end of the day, and we all joked.

'And I did all this research on Beelzebub, too,' Andrew said.

The oncologist corrected him gently. 'Bevacizumab.'

It was then that he told us that drug companies want the generic names to be impossible to remember.

'Although I've finally remembered temozolomide,' I said. 'Now that I am no longer on it.'

According to the oncologist, the person who discovered temozolomide died later of a brain tumour.

'And you know Georgia wrote a book that was just about to be published when she was diagnosed — a book in which the main character has a brain tumour,' Andrew said.

Andrew used to urge the oncologist to read my columns in *The Saturday Paper*, and I would tell him, don't — you don't want to read about brain cancer in your time off, I would say.

This time Andrew urged him to read my book. 'It's called *Between a Wolf and a Dog*,' he said.

The oncologist smiled. He was used to Andrew's support for my work, but we all knew he wasn't going to read it.

It is impossible for me to think of that book without feeling vertigo, a strange sense of peering down at myself from a great height. You see, I have always drawn on myself, on what I have experienced, in my writing. But I had never before predicted what was to come.

I started on *Between a Wolf and a Dog* about four years ago. It's hard to remember the kernel, the grit that began the

process, but I have a sense that I wanted simply to write about life — life from the middle and life from the end. The ordinary joys and sorrows that seem so momentous when you think you have all the time in the world, compared with how you view them when you know you're going to die.

I asked a doctor friend of mine for an illness. I told him I wanted one in which there was no hope.

'This character is pragmatic,' I said. 'She doesn't want to go through treatment if it is not going to cure her, if her time is limited. She wants to end her life on her own terms, while she is able.'

My friend suggested brain cancer.

'Perfect,' I said.

He was sketchy on the medical details (he was only a student at that time), and I decided my character would suffer from excruciating headaches. I didn't dream up an impairment to her language, or seizures, or loss of control of movement, which I know now are common to brain tumours.

As I was writing the first draft, Anne's behaviour was becoming increasingly worrying. Dates and appointment times, along with her finances, had gone — but she never had much of a grasp on numbers, as her vagueness with the value of that Tasmanian book demonstrated. Her sense of direction was also becoming worse. She frequently got lost, even driving to my place, and I would tell her to stay where she was and I'd come and find her. She never obeyed me, ringing me again from her mobile, from another street, sure that she was on the right track

now. The edits for her book on peace became impossible to wrangle, and her disposition, which was usually calm, became more and more erratic as she frequently lost her temper with me.

Anne had always said that she wanted to die, to be able to take her own life, if she had Alzheimer's. She had an advanced directive and pledges with various friends (I wouldn't ask you to put a pillow over my face, she would say, but I want to be able to end it). She didn't want to suffer like her own mother had, and she talked frequently of how her mother, who'd also had Alzheimer's, had gone into a home where she was strapped to a chair and was totally gaga, dosed up on drugs and stark raving mad. These are Anne's words, and her fear was genuine. I had known it since I was a child.

When she was diagnosed, on her 84th birthday, she was ashen. Not knowing the extent of her terror, the geriatrician didn't give her the news with the delicacy she needed. Perhaps there is no easy or right way to tell someone that they have dementia.

But in the weeks that followed her diagnosis, she never once talked of wanting to die.

In fact, she often said to me: 'I'm not going to kill myself'.

I had cold feet about publishing my book. Anne was still reading then, and she was always so proud of my work. Her emotional state was delicate. I didn't want her to conflate the older character in my book with herself, to think that I was wishing she would end it all.

I put off the publication.

GEORGIA BLAIN

The months progressed, with frequent doctors' appointments, small crisis after small crisis, and Anne deteriorated. In retrospect it was rapid, but it didn't feel so at the time.

As it became clear that she was no longer able to read, that the whole world of books and writing was no longer even on the periphery of her life, I turned to editing my novel in the brief snatches of time I had.

I completed the structural edit in a couple of months, and sent it back to my publishers.

There was to-ing and fro-ing as there always is with edits — a little bit more here, a further tuck there — but when I had just finished the first of the finer changes, I started getting calls about Rosie from her daughter.

The news rocked us all.

Rosie's family wanted to shield her from the diagnosis, to keep Rosie buoyant, and they asked her friends not to dwell on the illness too much when we were with her. Rosie, too, seemed to want to slide over any mention of the cancer.

In the middle of the night, I woke up, my heart beating loud, the sweat on my body cold.

I was going to be publishing a book with a central character who had brain cancer. The woman knew there was no cure.

I didn't know how to broach it with Rosie's family, if at all.

At that stage Rosie was still reading, and her command of language was better than it would later be. She regularly asked me about my work — when would it be published? Was I pleased with it?

I always gave her my manuscripts when they were in their final stages.

For the first time, I began lying to her; or perhaps it was more untruths by omission. There was so much that I couldn't talk to her about: the tumour, her treatment, or my work.

I thought that I could change the cancer in my book. Pancreatic, perhaps. It wouldn't be too hard. Perhaps it would even be better. I would weave out the headaches. I talked to a friend whose father had died of pancreatic cancer. She told me of his excruciating death in the corridors of the hospital, pleading for more morphine. My character would want to avoid that, I thought.

But in the end I talked to Rosie's daughter, feeling ashamed because I knew they had so much more to deal with than my book, but adamant I didn't want them to come to it unprepared, to see the reviews, to read it, to let Rosie read it.

She was taken aback.

'I'm sorry,' I kept saying. 'It is just one of those awful coincidences, and I just wanted you to know. I didn't want you to think that I was writing about Rosie.'

It was late October then.

She asked me when it was going to be published.

'April,' I told her.

I remember her words in response. 'That's a long time away,' she said. 'Who knows what will have happened by then.'

Less than a week later, I collapsed in the garden, on that bed of blossoms, my body jerking from the pressure in my brain,

caused by a tumour that in a matter of months had reached the size of a golf ball.

It is hard to believe. We often expect reality as we experience it to be less dramatic than fiction, and most of the time it is. But this was a perfect storm: a confluence of dark clouds gathering, all lined up in the horizon, every one of them heading my way.

Rosie has never read my book. It's the first novel of mine she hasn't read. Anne has never read it either. By the time it was published, neither of them were capable of reading. It's not as though I needed their approval, or their support — I have learnt to rely on my own judgement as to whether a piece of writing works — but it was a strange absence.

I remember Anne in particular used to go into bookshops and sneak copies of my novels onto the front shelves. She used to buy them for everyone she knew, here in Australia and back in England. Whenever a book of mine came out, her assistants would be busy, wrapping parcels for the post.

We form stories to make sense of what is happening to us. I do it with fiction and memoir. I now know that my last novel was very much informed by Anne's mortality. It was my love story to her — all the wash and grit and rubbish of life ultimately receding to a purer place.

If the plot line for *Between A Wolf and A Dog* had followed this last year of my life, I hope that my editor would have advised me to lose a cloud or two.

'The central character has just put her mother in a home with Alzheimer's, her mentor and best friend has terminal brain cancer,

she has written a book about terminal brain cancer, and now she has it, too,' she would have said. 'Maybe a little too much?'

I would have needed to be a far more skilful writer than I am to escape the criticisms of being overblown, or perhaps too fond of artifice; too young and with a tendency to the dramatic, labouring a point of some kind, perhaps about coincidence.

Yet, sometimes life is like that. The man who invented temozolomide died of a brain tumour. Each time I visit the oncologist, I go to the Chris O'Brien Lifehouse, named after the head and neck surgeon who was instrumental in raising funds for a building that is a state-of-the-art integrated cancer treatment centre. He, too, died of glioblastoma. And, dare I say it, but a year before this perfect storm gathered, I was brought on to help write copy for the Lifehouse, and I thought: *if I ever have cancer, what a place to go; it sounds amazing.*

Just after Odessa turned one, she started going to a small day-care centre on the edge of Tamarama and South Bondi.

She still had her afternoons at Anne's every Wednesday, but on Tuesday and Thursday we dropped her off after the early-morning rush, picking her up again as the afternoon sea breeze, stiff with salt, cooled down the heat of the day.

There was a baby's room, a toddler's room, and a room for the children that were going to school next year. She fell somewhere in between the first two. Not yet walking, she made her way around the centre on her hands and feet, a downward-dog pose that she used to get around at great speed. Unsteady on her legs, she still chanted 'Updown' each time she tried to get herself up, wanting to grasp a toy or a Little Golden Book that was just out of reach.

At the centre she never napped, but she would lie quietly, watchfully. One of the carers, who was particularly fond of her, soon took to putting books in her cot, and she would turn the pages, her voice murmuring, sing-song, just above a whisper,

nonsense words and coos of delight.

In the early evening, when she came home, she played out her day, always focusing on naptime. At first, we didn't realise what she was doing, but as the routine was regularly repeated, it became more obvious.

She took all the stuffed toys in her room — Lola and Lula, Mousie, Snowie, Henry, and the others whose names I've now forgotten — and laid them out on cushions and pillows. Carefully, she put a blanket over each of them, and when she ran out of blankets, a tissue, and she whispered 'night night' to all of them individually. Occasionally, she would have to stop on her rounds to tend to someone who was misbehaving, or who wanted another drink.

I don't think the baby Odessa was ever in the story. She was the adult, the one who had the power in her narrative of the day's events. Perhaps it was because she was troubled by naptime, as she couldn't sleep as she was meant to, or perhaps it was simply that this was the space in the day in which she was able to observe, at peace and uninterrupted.

As she became older, and we were able to walk her to the day-care centre, she would demand stories as a distraction. I was terrible at telling them, soon bored by the rambling nature of a tale that I was making up on the spot, and it didn't take long before she gave up on me, the pair of us slipping in and out of conversation and silence. But Andrew, who has always been the soft touch in our house, told her a story that continued day after day.

'Tell me the made-up story with bad witches,' she always said. And he would oblige.

When we all walked together it would frustrate me immensely, this tale that seemed to break every narrative structure, leaving half-finished plot lines behind us, characters who changed abruptly, scenarios that didn't make sense. Odessa loved it, partly because she had control over her parents during the walk, but this wasn't the entire reason. She liked the tale itself, and the fact that it defied every convention didn't diminish her enjoyment.

I was never formally schooled in how to build a story. Like most writers, I learnt by reading. But in the second trimester of my pregnancy with her, I went to a course in scriptwriting. I didn't want to be a scriptwriter, but I thought that maybe in the future I would want to try it, and I would have no time to study when I became a mother. (During this time, I also read *War and Peace*, *Anna Karenina*, and all of Dostoyevsky's novels, panicked that I would never be able to completely absorb myself in a book again once I had a child.)

The teacher was a Joseph Campbell devotee, and I became increasingly irritated by the way in which he felt all writing could be reduced to a simple formula.

He challenged us to name a script for a film that we'd recently seen that defied the hero's journey.

'I don't want something that just messes with the linear structure but still buys into the journey,' he said. 'I want something you have seen that that does not follow this trajectory in any way.'

I hated that I couldn't.

As a writer, I have found myself growing ever more frustrated by the need for plot. It often seems like a clanking piece of machinery dragging along behind me. What interests me more is mood, or character, or setting, and I want the plot to be woven in artfully, almost invisible, a narrative drive humming underneath, propelling us forward.

Naively, the first time I wrote about my life in *Births Deaths Marriages*, I thought that I would escape these shackles. Looking back, I find it strange that I had such a foolish expectation. Life is an amorphous mess, a huge soup of details that we wade our way through, and in order to make sense of what is happening to us, we impose structure, or narrative. It is inescapable.

Even Knausgård, who is endlessly distracted by the chaff and dust, mathematically structures his experiences within a larger whole — the story of becoming a writer, and, within a larger framework, the story of the modern ego, filled with a sense of its own importance. There are many ways he could tell this story, but this is the way he has chosen.

Before Joseph Campbell gave us the hero's journey, Vladimir Propp analysed many of Russia's folk tales and broke them down into thirty-one what he called narratemes, and the sequence in which they occur. While not all stories contain all of the narratemes, it is almost impossible to find fairytales or folk tales that contain none. Even Andrew's stories for Odessa contained many of them, though the order was jumbled, and any consistency of character and genre was frequently defied.

Now that I am nearing the end of my life, I have such an extraordinary plot at my disposal — one that needs to be made to look a little more haphazard to be believable, rather than being in need of shape (which is more usual with the stuff of life). Yet, I am resisting conventional structure more than ever.

I am in the third sphere of Propp's morphology, commonly called 'The Donor Sequence', twelve through to nineteen of the narratemes:

12. Testing: Hero is challenged to prove heroic qualities
13. Reaction: Hero responds to the test
14. Acquisition: Hero gains magical item
15. Guidance: Hero reaches destination
16. Struggle: Hero and villain do battle
17. Branding: Hero is branded
18. Victory: Villain is defeated
19. Initial misfortune or lack is resolved.

This is how most illness memoirs go — you fall ill, you prove your heroic qualities in the face of this challenge, you are treated and do battle with the illness, and the sickness is defeated, or you are defeated, but you have learnt what it is to live, and you have made peace with yourself and those around you.

I don't want to tell this tale. I have so many other stories to tell, and I hope to keep weaving words and language into intricate new structures, but sometimes I feel the lure of that subterranean current dragging me under, forcing me to tell the

story of my illness within this framework.

The archetypal myth that resonates with me above all others is Demeter's journey to rescue her daughter, Persephone, from the Underworld. In my first year of high school, I was awarded a prize for English Literature: a hardcover version of this tale with illustrations on every page. These were prints of watercolours: washed out ecru, charcoal, the pale pink of the shades, the deep green of the cypress, the ghostly mauve of an owl, and the lurid red of the pomegranate seeds. At the time, I thought these were exquisite; now, I think they are ugly — but I still have this book on my shelves.

Persephone is the daughter of Zeus and Demeter, the Ruler of the Gods and the Goddess of the Grain and the Harvest respectively. When Persephone is stolen by Hades, the God of the Underworld, Demeter rages across the earth, searching for her daughter. No crops will grow, and the world is plunged into winter.

There are many versions, as there are with all Greek myths, some with Zeus telling Demeter that Hades has stolen her daughter, some with Helios revealing the truth.

Demeter goes to the Underworld to bring Persephone back, but just as she is about to return with her, a single shade blocks her path. Apparently, Persephone has eaten six pomegranate seeds while she was with Hades, and to eat the food of her captor means that she has to remain with her captor.

I remember that moment in my version of the tale: Hades asking if Persephone has eaten anything and her stating that

she has not, but the illustration showing us Persephone's fingers crossed behind her back. Turn the page and there is that damn shade, piping up in his reedy, horrible voice that she is a liar. 'I saw Persephone eat six pomegranate seeds.'

Let it go, I wanted to tell him. *Just let it go.*

But no, he couldn't.

In my version, Demeter returns to the earth and her rage knows no end. Everyone is starving, and Zeus has to intervene.

For every pomegranate seed Persephone has eaten, she will remain a month of each year. This is autumn and winter. But when she returns, spring with its blossoms and new growth comes with her.

Sometimes, I like to imagine my illness cast within the structure of this tale. As I collapsed onto that bed of blossoms, lilac and coral-red, the Underworld opened up beneath me and I was plunged into darkness. What happened when I was out cold with the seizure? Was that what death is like?

Now that I have lived with the shades, there is always a part of me that remains in Hades. I have seen it, and I will return.

There are times when I think Anne is already dwelling there. When I walk into her room in the nursing home, she often appears to be dead. Her face is immobile, her skin dry, her eyes are closed, and her mouth is open, but she doesn't seem to be breathing. And then she starts, a great gasp of air filling her lungs.

Perhaps she has been there with Hades bargaining for my return to the living. Because it is wrong for a daughter to die before a mother. *Take me*, she would say.

I know this is foolish. She is completely trapped within the prism of her own illness and has little awareness of my cancer, despite the fact that we have told her often, explaining why I cannot come to see her as often as I would like.

Sometimes, she takes it in. Sometimes, she doesn't.

'Are you better?' she asks occasionally.

But most of the time she is in her own boat, journeying across the River Styx, a journey that has nothing to do with me.

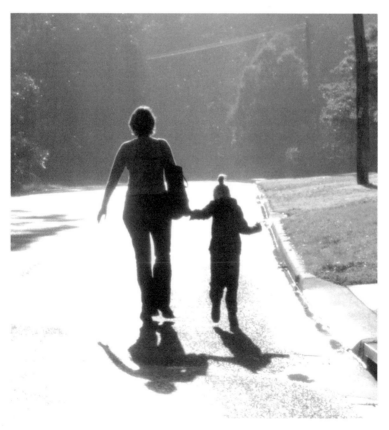

Georgia and Odessa, c. 2003

When she was learning French, Odessa told me that generally adjectives come after the noun. However, as with all rules in language, there are exceptions, and these can be grouped under the acronym BAGS — adjectives that describe Beauty, Age, Goodness, and Size. These are even more loosely referred to as adjectives that express an opinion, rather than a fact.

And then these exceptions themselves have numerous tweaks, with some adjectives able to be placed before or after a word, altering the meaning. For example, *pauvre* means wretched if it's before the noun, and poor (as in not rich) if it's after the noun. Although poor could surely be a matter of opinion in both senses of the word, as it depends on the point of view of the speaker and his or her position in life.

However, the point is that these are the rules (and exceptions to those rules) that you have to learn if you are not a native speaker, whereas if you are speaking in your first language, it seems as if you can learn your way around these rules by a process akin to osmosis.

I was surprised to learn that there is an order to our placement of adjectives in English. The first is always opinion, followed by size, age, shape, colour, origin, material, and purpose — all of which precede the noun. Odessa disputes how hard and fast this rule is; her Latin teacher said the order is a matter of going from the general to the particular, like a wide funnel. Nevertheless, I am sipping coffee out of a small, seventies, brown, china mug as I write. If I said I had my coffee in a seventies, small, china, brown mug, you might think that I was not an English speaker or that there was something wrong with my speech.

When you teach writing, you tell students to be wary of adjectives and adverbs, to prune them assiduously. And, as you edit your work, to keep pruning, with an eye to exactitude. Do you really need that word, and if you need it, is it the right word?

With memoir particularly, you want precision. Each word has to be carefully chosen. A friend, who is an editor, once said the editing process is akin to stripping your work of all colour and then adding in hues, carefully, subtly, with an eye on the whole.

We have so many words that are similar in meaning, their differences slight, a curl of wood shaving all that separates them.

Each morning I do a meditation in a high-backed, orange, Danish armchair (I couldn't resist). I usually get up before Andrew and Odessa, turning on the heater on cool mornings, and waking up the dog, whose tail always thumps in delight at the first sign of human company after a long, lonely night.

I have an App that has various guided meditations on it, packages that are all very similar, but which are loosely grouped

under headings like 'Patience' or 'Stress'.

The last I did was a series of ten on 'Kindness'.

Each one is accompanied by a short introductory talk, and each time, as I settle back in the chair, I swear to myself that I will pay attention to this talk, I will focus — but invariably I drift off, much to my shame. However, with the first talk on kindness, I listened, perhaps for the wrong reason. It was about the difference between kindness and compassion. Do those words mean different things? Is compassion more a desire to ease suffering in others, whereas kindness has less of a need for suffering as a prerequisite? Can you be kind without being compassionate — or compassionate without being kind? I don't think the latter is possible, but the former might be.

We don't often think about these nuances in words, or at least not consciously, but we make our way around this gorgeous paint box of so many different hues, selecting subtly different colours with dexterity and art. It is a marvel. Yet, if you are forced to think about what you're doing — as I have to do when I become tired — it stops making sense, and language becomes a clumsy tool.

Hearing this in myself is hard, and witnessing it in my writing is also difficult, but I have learnt the boundaries of the paddock (while also knowing that they may shrink). I can ride out for about three quarters of an hour, under optimal circumstances, before I have to stop and rest. I need silence before I can head for home again.

I often think of Rosie, who is only capable of very short

rides, each one getting shorter and shorter. I assume it frustrates her immensely, and sometimes when I see her, I witness it.

Immediately after my diagnosis, Rosie and I were travelling near each other. She was slightly ahead of me in treatment at first. We would occasionally bump into each other in the radiation clinic, both of us losing our hair, both of us tired, each of us just holding the other's hand, not talking too much, but knowing what the other was going through. I remember when she finished her last radiation session, and how envious I was. I had to go beyond the Christmas break.

Even then, in the clinic, we didn't speak of the illness. I still don't know if she wanted to — I don't think she did — but as her language became worse, it became more difficult, even if she had wanted to discuss it. Her tumour was larger than mine and the operation didn't remove all of it. She also had a lot of swelling in the brain, perhaps caused by the surgery or the radiation, or both.

It wasn't long before our tracks separated. She went downhill, and it was hard to witness. I felt for her and I was afraid for myself. *Why?* I would often think. *Why is this happening? It's cruel to have her showing me the way.*

Odessa and I once joked about how I had obviously angered some god somewhere, at some time, and even though it would give some comfort to think that there was a reason — that perhaps I could atone — there isn't. If there are gods, they are capricious and their motives are unfathomable. This is life, as I frequently remind myself. This is life.

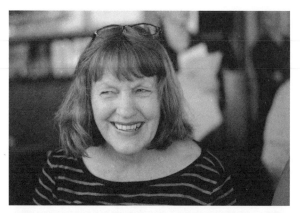

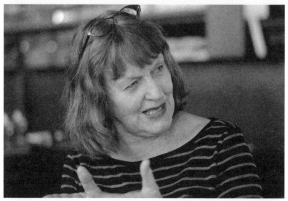

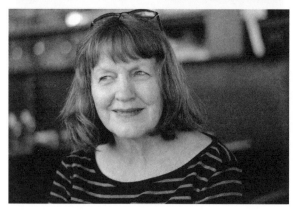

Rosie Scott, Glebe restaurant, August 2014

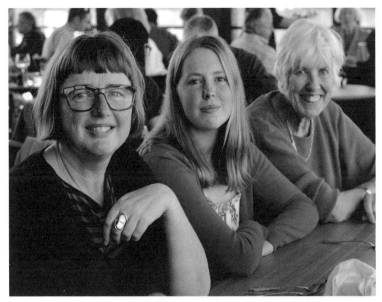

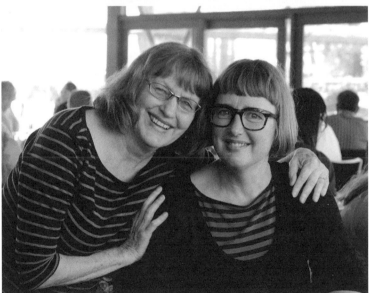

Above: Georgia, Odessa, and Anne, Glebe restaurant, August 2014
Below: Rosie and Georgia, Glebe restaurant, August 2014

I used to ring Rosie every fortnight or so, but our conversations became more difficult. In the past, before we became ill, we had often talked for well over an hour on the phone. Fluid, quicksilver, mercurial talks that would skip lightly from topic to topic.

Perhaps it would have been easier if we'd Skyped, so that I could see her expression, but I was never great at technology, and she was even worse. I had to rely on her husband, Danny, and her daughters to be on the phone with her, translating for both of us, always cheerful, despite how hard it must have been for them.

Recently, just before she went into palliative care, Danny brought her over to visit us. We sat around the kitchen table talking, and although Rosie couldn't say much, her presence in the conversation was strong.

It was her nouns, Danny said at one stage, turning to Rosie and holding her hand. That was what she had most difficulty with.

The building blocks. The first words we often express when we learn a language. The things we need or desire, the objects we want to alert another to; and when we first begin to speak, we often accompany those words by pointing. If the nouns are gone, it's impossible. These are the words on which we hang all other words.

He talked about how hard it was for Rosie to express what she was going through. Strangely, this was the first time this had occurred to me. Most of the time, I had assumed she didn't

want to talk because talking of the illness made her stressed, just as talking of arrangements made me tongue-tied.

Danny had thought hypnotherapy would help — a non-verbal way of alleviating (and I am dubious about my use of that word — perhaps 'expressing' is more apt) the experience of this illness. He had tried it himself and he had liked it.

Early on in my own treatment, I had been to see a counsellor, and I was struck by how futile, how puny my words were in the face of this illness. I didn't know why I was there — because I felt I should be, I suppose. There was no comfort that could be given. And then I realised it was nothing more than an allotted hour in which I could grieve and express my fears, and that that was enough. At the end of the sixty minutes, I dried my eyes, cleaned my glasses, and went out to face the world again.

As the breakdown in Rosie's language affected her capacity to write as well, there was no way in which she could put her fears into words. Sometimes, I wondered whether Rosie would be able to draw what she meant, but I didn't ask. I think the two (the written word and the picture) would be inextricably linked.

I remember we used to play a game called Pictionary, where we had to illustrate phrases or words, like a game of charades with pen and paper. Being able to guess what your teammate was drawing, and what it meant, was contingent on how well and quickly he or she could draw. But it helped if you knew that person well, if you knew the associations that certain phrases would bring up.

Once, I played it with Anne, and it was so easy for me to

guess. She drew a picture of duck à l'orange (how I even knew it *was* that is something I still marvel at, particularly as she was terrible at drawing). She was illustrating the phrase 'duck for cover', and as soon as she drew the lid on the casserole dish, I knew what it was. The associations, the links in the chain that led from one to the other, the message transmitted from her to me were all so quickly discerned. Just as when I go into the nursing home and she is rambling, agitated, sure that she is in trouble, that no one likes her, that her hands are dirty, I can quickly surmise what has happened that morning.

It's also like that when Rosie, unable to speak, would beam in delight on greeting me and then stroke the side of my cheek with tenderness and compassion (and kindness is not the right word), transmitting so much love and care and empathy without words.

Many people say we only have one story in us, and we write it out again and again. We dress it up in different plots and genres, trying on new clothes, examining it from new angles, but essentially, it is the same.

I no longer apologise for this. Mine has always been about family, or lack of: the absent father, mother, and sibling, whether through death, obsession with work; the hand grenade that is jettisoned into this unit, atomising each of the members.

Each time I write this story, I examine it from a fresh wealth of experiences, the stage where I am at in life. I know that as I have got older, and perhaps more forgiving and understanding of people's foibles and weaknesses, I have allowed more room for the presence of love and forgiveness.

Anne is always central to my stories — or perhaps it would be more accurate to say the mother role plays a big part in my fiction and memoir.

I only ever met Anne's mother, Barbara, once, when I was too young to remember. Anne loved her, but she also talked

about how Barbara, like her and myself, didn't take easily to being a mother. Anne was brought up by a formidable nanny with a capacious bosom.

When we were cleaning out Anne's house, we found a recording of Barbara, which a friend has since digitised for us. Barbara was living in London, and had just put Anne on the train, the first leg of a long sea voyage to Australia, where she would be joining Ellis, my father, ultimately to marry him and have their three children.

I'm not sure of the background to this recording. It was a voice letter from Barbara to Ellis about Anne's departure. I think she spoke to him rather than Anne herself because this was an era in which communication to women was mediated through the men in their lives. Perhaps it was also Ellis's reel-to-reel machine (he was a radio interviewer for the ABC at the time), although I find it strange that he would have left a recorder behind in London. Maybe it was Anne's equipment. She termed herself a journalist at this stage in her life, and perhaps she had bought a new recorder for her journey.

Barbara was nervous about speaking into a microphone — she felt 'rather silly', she said over and over again. She described shopping for Anne's trousseau — 'you will have quite the ravishing bride,' she repeated frequently — and the emotion she felt on saying goodbye to her daughter: 'I had to have a few brandy and sodas, and a cigarette.'

But the predominant sense that came through that recording was the trepidation she felt on letting her daughter go to the

other side of the world to marry a man who was much older than her, had already had a wife, and, above all, whom she didn't like.

'You will be happy, Ellis,' she said, and this phrase was repeated more than any other on the recording, a fervent wish rather than a question or command.

Listening to it through my computer, Andrew and I cried. It was partly just hearing a disembodied voice from another era, so crisp and present, the beginning of Anne's story as I had known it. It was also because my mother had talked so much about her mother in the last months, the horror she had felt at seeing her in a nursing home with Alzheimer's and being able to do nothing. Anne lived in Australia, and Barbara lived in London.

However, more than anything, it was that I knew how this story played out. Barbara was right to feel trepidation. Ellis was possessive, domineering, paranoid, and obsessive-compulsive. He was also physically abusive. And it took Anne sixteen years to leave him.

This was the fodder for so much of my writing. I fed off it, over and over again.

But as I came to understand why it was so hard for Anne to leave, and as I built my own life with Andrew and Odessa, the story began to play out in different ways. The light came in, just faint and intermittent at first, and then stronger.

We tried to play Anne an extract of this recording of her mother's voice a few months ago. She loved her mother, and we thought it would soothe her to hear her again. But it only

agitated her. She didn't understand how her voice could be on the machine, despite her having no concept of time, no concept of who has gone and who is still with us.

I've learnt that the best thing to do is tell her that I love her and sit in silence holding her hand. There is not much more that I can do. I have few regrets, but I wish I had told her that more often in the past.

I know that I have limited time.

Last week I had another seizure, just before the blossoms came out. It was ten months after the first time I collapsed on that carpet of lilac and coral-red. But this time I wasn't in my garden; I was at a friend's house. I was conscious for most of it and I was terrified. All of me fought to keep breathing. I tried to still myself, but I was in a tunnel, powerless, life in its busyness so very distant, voices talking about ambulances, telling me I was okay, Andrew holding me.

I spent the day back in the hospital where I began, being scanned again, hearing bad news again. The little I have read (and I avoid reading about this illness) tells me that this is the beginning of the decline. That brief window of no medical intervention was very brief.

And so here we are: Rosie, Anne, and me.

I would like to end this with the three of us alive. Anne and Rosie have little ability to communicate, but they have given me so much; a lifeline that I will keep scrambling up until I can do it no more. And I am hoping that I will still be capable of the invisible work: the editing. I know this requires a surgical

THE MUSEUM OF WORDS

precision with language that is feeling more and more out of my grasp, but I will stretch and reach for the right tenses, the clauses, the overarching structure to form a precise but shimmering picture of what I want to represent. This miniature is my life in words, and I have been so grateful for every minute of it.

Image credits

All photos © Andrew G Taylor except:

pp 17   Georgia 1971, Ellis Blain

pp 22   Anne and Georgia, 1971 Ellis Blain

pp 71   Anne and Gough Whitlam, unknown

          Anne in 2GB studios, unknown

pp 91   Andrew and Odessa reading, Georgia Blain

pp 106   View from Bondi flat, Georgia Blain

pp 119   Sari and Anne in workroom, Sari Braithwaite and

          Carolyn Constantine.

pp 122   Empty bookshelves, Georgia Blain

THE MUSEUM
OF WORDS

a

memoir

of

language,

writing,

and

mortality

Georgia Blain

SCRIBE

Melbourne • London